Anticipating and Assessing Health Care Technology Volume 8

Scenario Commission on Future
Health Care Technology

chairman H. David Banta

senior researcher Dr. ir. W.T. van Beekum

Anticipating and Assessing Health Care Technology Volume 8

Potentials for Home Care Technology

A report, commissioned by the
Steering Committee on Future Health Scenarios

1988
Kluwer Academic Publishers
Dordrecht – Boston – London

Distributors

for the United States and Canada: Kluwer Academic Publishers.
101 Philip Drive, Norwell, MA 02061, U.S.A.
For all other countries: Kluwer Academic Publishers Group,
P.O. Box 322, 3300 AH Dordrecht, The Netherlands

Steering Committee
on Future Health Scenarios
P.O. Box 5406
2280 HK Rijswijk
The Netherlands
Telephone: 070-407209

ISBN-13: 978-94-010-7092-8 e-ISBN-13: 978-94-009-1329-5
DOI: 10.1007/978-94-009-1329-5

Foreword

This report, **Potentials for Home Care Technology**, is the eighth report from the STG Commission on Future Health Care Technology and one of a series of case studies from that project. The STG (Stuurgroep Toekomstscenario's Gezondheidzorg) was established in 1983 as an independent advisory group to the State Secretary for Welfare, Public Health, and Cultural Affairs (WVC) to assist in long-range health planning efforts. Thus far, STG commissions have examined cardiovascular disease, cancer, aging, and life styles as issues of importance to the health of the Dutch population in the future.

Obviously, health care technology is of great concern to the government. On the one hand, technology is one of the major tools to promote a healthy population. On the other hand, the costs of health care have been rising at an alarming rate in recent years. These two facts, along with the social consequences of certain technologies such as genetic screening, led the STG to establish the Commission on Future Health Care Technology in 1985. The European Office of the World Health Organization (EURO) cosponsored the project. The Health Council (Gezondheidsraad) agreed to cooperate with the project by furnishing space and intellectual and logistical support.

The goal of the Commission's work is to develop sufficient information on future technological developments in health and health care to assist planning for their consequences.

The first report, **Anticipating and Assessing Health Care Technology**, gave the overall context for activities concerning future health care technology. The government and Dutch society as a whole must move rapidly to deal with the consequences of technological change in health care. The first report provided conclusions for achieving this purpose, focusing on the need to develop a national program or system of health care technology assessment.

The second report, **Future Technological Changes**, presented detailed information on anticipated future health care technologies. In the context of STG's studies, this might be considered an 'early warning system' for health care technology.

The third report, **Developments in the Regeneration, Repair and Reorganization of Nervous Tissue**, focused on future applications of neurosciences, especially regarding Alzheimer's disease, Parkinson's disease, and accidents involving nervous system trauma.

The fourth report, **Health Care Applications of Lasers: The Future Treatment of Coronary Artery Disease«MDNM»**, presents a general introduction to lasers in health care, although more detailed information is presented in Volume II. The main purpose of this case study is to examine the possible impacts of one application of lasers: the treatment of coronary artery disease.

The fifth report, **Developments in Genetic Testing**, examines another application of the new biotechnology, the rapidly developing field of genetics. The genetic revolution has now truly begun and it will transform the ways that society deals with its genetic inheritance. The implications of this new technology are far-reaching. The report explores some of these implications and suggests the importance of careful monitoring of this field.

The sixth report, **Applications of the New Biotechnology: The Case of Vaccines**, discusses developments in the new biotechnology. The ability to directly manipulate the genetic structure of organisms has lead to dramatic changes in biological research, and is now beginning to transform practical technology as well. The report presents some of the new developments in diagnostic and therapeutic technologies. The main purpose of the report, however, is to point out the potential applications in vaccine development and possible future impacts of this field on the health of the Netherlands population.

The seventh report, **Computer Assisted Medical Imaging: The Case of Picture Archiving and Communications Systems (PACS)**, presents information on an important new technology. Since the early 1970s, departments of radiology have gradually turned to imaging with computers, and there are now predictions that all medical images, including conventional x-rays, will be computerized. Such a move would have great potential advantages, but the costs to the health care system and society would also be large. It is important for Dutch society to become aware of these developments and to determine the best course of future action.

This report, the final one from the project on future health care technology, **Potentials for Home Care Technology**, gives an overview of present and future developments in an important and often-neglected field of health care. The report also describes and analyses the home care system of the Netherlands, and concludes that the home care system is not structured to be receptive to technology. Therefore, the report suggests ways that the home care system could be improved.

As Chairman of the STG, I am delighted to present this report, and I thank the Commission very sincerely for its rapid and excellent work. The government expects to see changes in policies toward health care technology, and I am certain that the report will be a substantial help in that process of change.

The report was prepared by the Commission's staff, which is listed in this report. The staff was led by Dr. David Banta, an American who agreed to spend two years with the STG chairing the Commission. The decision to invite Dr. Banta to the Netherlands was a recognition of the international nature of issues concerning health care technology. I would also like to point out the presence of a Swede, Dr. Henry Danielsson, and a Belgian, Professor Jan Blanpain, on the Commission. Dr. Johannes Vang from WHO/EURO was an official observer on the Commission. We are particularly grateful to these outside guests.

The reports have been developed with the help of experts and reviewed by the Commission and by many other individuals and groups representing a wide range of disciplines and perspectives. We are grateful for their many contributions. As with all STG reports, however, the content of the report is the responsibility of the Commission and the STG and does not necessarily represent the position of any of those who assisted or of the Ministry of WVC.

J. van Londen
Chairman, STG

Preface

As noted in the Foreword, this report is one of several volumes resulting from this study of future health care technology.

The purpose of the study, as formulated by the STG, was to analyze future health care technology. Part of the task was to develop an 'early warning system' for health care technology. The primary goal of the project was to develop a list or description of a number of possible and probable future health care technologies, as well as information on their importance. Within the limits of time and money, this has been done. However, given the vast number of possible future health care technologies, complete information on the importance of each area could not be developed in any depth for all technology.

Therefore, four specific technologies were chosen and were prospectively assessed. These future technologies were examined in more depth, looking particularly at their future health and policy implications. Subsequently, the project was extended to September 1987, and two additional technologies were chosen for assessment.

The total output of the project is as follows:

Volume 1. GENERAL CONSIDERATIONS AND POLICY RECOMMENDATIONS

Volume 2. FUTURE TECHNOLOGICAL CHANGES

Volume 3. DEVELOPMENTS IN THE REGENERATION, REPAIR AND REORGANIZATION OF NERVOUS TISSUE

Volume 4. HEALTH CARE APPLICATIONS OF LASERS: THE FUTURE TREATMENT OF CORONARY ARTERY DISEASE

Volume 5. DEVELOPMENTS IN GENETIC TESTING

Volume 6. APPLICATIONS OF THE NEW BIOTECHNOLOGY: The Case of Vaccines

Volume 7. COMPUTER-ASSISTED MEDICAL IMAGING: The Case of Picture Archiving and Communications Systems (PACS)

Volume 8. POTENTIALS FOR HOME CARE TECHNOLOGY

The first report was addressed to an important purpose. The Commission reached the tentative conclusion early in its deliberations that a system for identifying future health care technology would be of limited benefit on its own. The Netherlands does not have an organized system for technology assessment in health care, and therefore information on the benefits, risks, financial costs, and social implications of technology is not available for new or established technology, generally speaking. The Commission saw the need for such a system. Studies aimed at the identification and assessment of future health care technologies must be developed within such a context, the Commission concluded. Therefore, Volume I was developed as an overall policy document, and contains summary material on future technologies.

The second report presented overall information on future health care technology. The report was based on information obtained from surveys done in the United States and in Europe.

The case studies are intended to examine important areas of future (and emerging) health care technology. However, many other potential subjects and applications could be examined. This case study, then, is only an example of what may be possible in evaluating the impacts of future health care technology.
Technological developments in health care are occurring rapidly, and the information on future technologies in these reports will rapidly become out-of-date. The Commission is aware of this fact, and hopes that it will be possible to continue an 'early warning system' that will periodically update such information and assess specific technologies.

The Ministry of Economical Affairs (EZ) supported the development of this case study because of the potential for industrial development in home care technology. Therefore, one of the central questions in this study is how to encourage industry to become more active in this area. Dr.ir. van Beekum, who worked on this study, also chairs a group sponsored by EZ on home care technology. To prevent duplication, it was decided that this report should focus on the home care system itself, while the other group would devote more attention to individual technologies.

This report is primarily addressed to policy makers and to those who are interested in national level policy making. At the same time, the Commission believes that the information in this report is an important basis for future activities in health care technology assessment in Netherlands and in other countries. The decisions called for in the policy conclusions are far-reaching, and raise a number of social, ethical, and cultural issues that are not dealt with in this report. Obviously, attempts to put the conclusions into operation would entail careful consideration of such issues.

Dr. H. David Banta
Chairman
Commission on Future Health Care Technology

Table of Contents

List of Technology Briefs

List of Tables

List of Figures

Introduction

Home health care is becoming a visible and much-discussed issue in countries such as the Netherlands. In general, home health care means the provision of health care services in the patient's home rather than an institutional setting or a provider's office (4;130). While successful home care often must involve a complex infrastructure of services, such as meals on wheels, remote shopping, mail delivery, and even possibly architecture of the home and design of transportation systems, this report focuses on organized health care services in the home, including services for the disabled. The term 'home care' in this report, then, may be considered to mean 'home health care'. Interest in home care is increasing as expenditures for health care are being limited (143). The aging of the population means that the needs for care will increase during the next decades. Home health care is often seen as offering the possibility of providing more services without greatly increasing the costs of the system of health care.

There seems little doubt that bringing health care services to people in their own homes can prevent hospitalization and institutionalization in nursing homes (15;19;108). People can also be discharged from the hospital sooner (4). The development of home care services can vastly enhance the quality of life of those who receive care (152).

Home care does not work as an alternative to institutionalization, however, unless a wide range of services, both medical and social, are available (92;143). The problems that must be dealt with are not simple ones, nor are they necessarily strictly medical. As people age, they become more frail and may require help in activities of daily living (98;109). People with physical or mental handicaps may need little in the way of medical care, but they can have problems of functioning. Often, families provide quite a lot of care, but they need the support of specialized providers and periodic relief from the burdens of day-to-day care.

Technological possibilities to support home care are expanding rapidly. Technology[1] used in home care includes medical technology, such as dialysis machines, respirators, insulin pumps, and devices to deliver cancer chemotherapy. Health care can also include devices to assist personal functions, including moving, reaching, preparing meals, and using the toilet. Finally, home care technology includes computers and telecommunications to support people in the home, to monitor their physical states, and to allow them to communicate easily with others, including health care providers.

What is the potential contribution of new and future developments in modern technology to developing home care systems? One fact is clear: the most important aspect of home care is indeed **care**, so one must look for different types of technology and a different role for technology than would be found in health care institutions such as hospitals. Home care services are people-intensive, and they will continue to be. Social supports and social contacts may often be the most critical part of home care. The question, then, is how can technology such as devices and prosthetics support or enhance these services (14)? How can such technology improve the quality of people's lives? And can it be done in a cost-effective manner?

If new and future technology is to make a substantial contribution to home care, it must be incorporated into a system of care. Home health care, however, has not been planned and developed systematically, but instead has grown incrementally to meet obvious needs. A true system of home care would include an identifiable array of interrelated and interacting components (32). There is, in this sense, no real home care system in the Netherlands, but instead a set of uncoordinated services. To implement new technology requires a supporting system. Technology must be developed in accordance with needs; it must be provided when appropriate; it must be paid for; it must be evaluated. The present-day organizations involved in home care do not seem able to take on these tasks.

Without a clearly organized system, industry also may not be able to identify a market for its technology.

---

[1]) Health care technology in this report includes the drugs, devices, and procedures used in health care and the organizational and supportive systems within which such care is delivered.

Planning a home care system would require the following steps (241):

1. stating the policy and broad goals;
2 gathering data to guide the planning process, including data on services available and needs that should be met;
3. identifying the priority health problems;
4. making major alternative proposals (including financial estimates);
5. developing a detailed plan with targets and standards;
6. implementing the plan; and
7. evaluating the effects of the plan and its implementation.

As described in this report, little data on home care in the Netherlands is available. Little is known about what people need or want. Still, a start can be made on developing a true system of home care.

This report, then, focuses on the system of home care, and not technology itself. The report starts from the assumption that complex technology **can** be a valuable part of home care, but that its role is severely limited without developments in the home care system itself. The report also presents examples of new and future technologies that could be beneficial in home care. The policy conclusions deal with possible changes in this system, as well as changes related to the technology of care.

The **organization** of the report is as follows: Part I of the report is made up of two sections. The first section gives a general background on home care services. The second section describes and critiques the approach to home care in the Netherlands. Part II of the report is divided into four sections that describe different types of technology that are presently used in home care and some future technologies that might be used in the future. The final section presents conclusions addressed to policies concerning home care.

Part I – General Issues in Home Care

Home health care means the provision of health care services in the patient's home rather than an institutional setting or a provider's office. Health care in this definition is rather broadly conceived, to include medical services provided by physicians, but also other services related to health, including rehabilitation, support for those with chronic illness or disability, and terminal care. The report focuses on such services because the major part of expenditures in health care are devoted to adults with acute and chronic illnesses and because modern technology seems to have the most to offer to this group.

The first section gives a general background on home care that may be applied to many countries.

The second section describes the specific situation of the Netherlands in home health care. While many of the generalizations in the previous Section apply to the Netherlands, not all do. The Netherlands also has its own specific problems and orientations. This section could be seen as a case study of the Netherlands, in the context of international developments in home care and home care technology.

An important part of home care in the Netherlands is home birth and infant care, involving (especially) midwives and nurses. This report focuses on chronically ill, disabled, and elderly people. The role of modern technology is limited in home birth as well as in infant care. For these reasons, home birth and infant care will not be described in any detail in this report.

Section 1 – Home care

Historical Perspective

Home care has always been an important part of health care. Traditionally, care was focused on the home or community. Hospitals were usually seen as places for the poor to go when they were too sick to care for themselves; they were essentially death houses. The hospital changed about 1900 with developments in medical technology, particularly with hospital hygiene, asepsis, and surgical anesthesia. With the development of vaccines and antibiotics, and the corresponding control of infectious diseases, the hospital role shifted toward care of people with chronic degenerative and neoplastic diseases (cancer). Now, more than 95 percent of people admitted to the hospital can expect to be discharged alive (81).

Economic, social, and cultural currents have greatly influenced such changes. The development of social insurance to pay for health care is one important example. Western society values scientific and technological knowledge, and people tend to seek medical assistance for more and more conditions. At the same time, recent research has begun to elucidate social, behavioral, and environmental factors in health and disease, and has led to consideration of a more ecological approach to health (67). This cultural shift will probably encourage more home care in the future.

Although attention in this century has shifted to the hospital, it should be borne in mind that most health related problems are still dealt within the home. Still, physicians became increasingly reluctant to make home visits and services for people in the home have not developed rapidly (26).

The recent attention to home care by policy makers is probably largely attributable to the problem of rising costs of health and social services (15). The increasing needs for care of the chronically ill, especially in light of an aging population (236), have put pressure on hospitals at a time that the number of hospital beds is being reduced. The health care system looks to home care as an alternative to meet these increasing needs. The home is also better able to house such services than in the past, with improved sanitary conditions, general availability of electricity for motors, the presence of telephones for access to professional help in emergencies, and availability of private and public transport (26).

General Considerations in Home Care

Home care is best seen as part of a continuum of comprehensive health care. Services must be appropriate to the needs of the patient. Persons needing home care may be acutely or chronically ill; their clinical conditions may range from clearly defined instabilities, physical or mental, to stabilized levels in need of continued supervision and maintenance. The level of need may range from total dependence to virtual independence (15).

Although home care has gained attention primarily as a method of controlling costs, its real value lies in improving quality and acceptability of care. In many cases, and especially when the problem is not an acute medical condition, the relationship between the provider and the patient may play an extremely important part in the healing and care process. The relationship is more equal and less 'medical' in the home setting. The provider may gain valuable information from visiting the home, especially in view of the fact that the home is the real setting of care during most of the time. In addition, many people with chronic illnesses would rather be at home than in the hospital or other institution. Home care thus may improve the quality of life of people with illness or disability (248;258).

Home care can also promote autonomy of people with illness or disability. Some observers predict a growing amount of dependency due to the aging of the population. However, dependency is a social state that can be altered through social and economic policies such as those related to age of retirement and distribution of resources between different age groups and social classes (149). Home care and further technological innovation, likewise, can make a contribution to minimizing dependency of those receiving care.

Although home care is the subject of an ever-growing literature, and is increasingly discussed in policy documents and conferences, it has not yet been effectively developed in the Netherlands or other countries. Home care has been hampered in general by a number of factors, including (26):

1. Wide variations in reimbursement. In general, reimbursement for older technologies is more favorable than that for newer technologies.
2. Financial incentives conspire against home care. Positive financial incentives are often lacking, and movement of services out of hospitals often leads to financial losses for physicians, hospitals, pharmacists, and patients themselves.
3. In many countries, home care is controlled by specialists or by hospital services.
4. In most countries, the health care system is, by its nature and because of its history, pro-institutional.

One danger in home care is that policy makers sometimes look to family and especially female relatives to provide an increasing amount of care for their relatives (65;124;191). Families, particularly female relatives, already provide a great deal of such care. A study in Britain found that the average time families spent caring for severely disabled elderly relatives was 3 hours 24 minutes a day, of which 3 hours 11 minutes was attributed to women and 13 minutes to men (176). It seems unlikely that families will take on a greatly increased burden. Present trends also show that more and more aged people are caring for other aged people; this particularly applies to spouses caring for each other (149). A goal for policy might be to maintain the present level of home care by giving support and relief to family members providing such care now. Further, it might be possible to find innovative new arrangements (such as paying elderly people for care given) that could expand such services. At the present, delivering home health care services is not very well paid and is generally a low-status activity. This problem, too, could be addressed by public policy measures.

An aspect of home health care that has received little attention is self-care (35;36;256). People with chronic illness and disability can often take care of themselves quite well after education and with some assistance from a professional. For example, people with diabetes mellitus are taking on increasing responsibility for their own treatment. Technological developments such as tests for urine or blood sugar and insulin pumps have encouraged such trends. As for the elderly, the majority do not need very much in the way of health and social services; the bulk of their care is self-care (249).

An aspect of home care particularly important for the elderly is social support. Social isolation is particularly prevalent among the elderly (249).

Most home care is given by informal networks of lay people, but special needs arise when no informal network is available, when informal carers are temporarily not available (illness, holiday), or when the situation of the patient demands professional care. Somewhere between informal care by relatives and neighbours and professional care is voluntary care by general organizations, such as meals on wheels, or by organizations of people suffering from particular diseases.

In cases where the informal network is not available or insufficiently supportive, available care seems to be given by professionals. However, some amount of informal care seems to be a condition for professional home care; if no informal care is available, admission to an old people's home or nursing home or a prolonged hospital stay is often necessary. On the other hand, particularly for chronically ill and handicapped people, professional home care relieves the informal carers temporarily from their burdens and helps them to continue in this role.

Professional home care services in general are fragmented, uncoordinated, and available through different programs with different admission standards and different requirements for continuing in the program. Often, only those who can afford to pay themselves, or those living in certain geographic areas are able to obtain care in the home. A pressing need in the future is to develop a true system for home care with universal access as part of the health care system. An important part of a system is to have a clear definition of which person or organization can prescribe or order services for an individual (15;186).

Training of health care providers to meet certain needs is an important consideration. For example, diabetes is a relatively prevalent condition in the typical general practitioner's office, with about 50 patients per practice. Diabetes can be a difficult problem, and special training of the clinician may be needed. Training for handling this condition seems important. However, it is not possible to train the clinician to deal with every problem. Therefore, the focus should be on more prevalent conditions.

Needs for Home Care

Although every person sometimes needs home care, e.g., in episodes of acute illness, a number of population groups may be identified who more or less depend on home care for their functioning in the community. The most important population groups with special needs for home care include:

- chronically ill people;
- elderly people, who (depending on their functional status) are more or less dependent of informal and professional carers;
- people who are discharged from the hospital;
- mentally and/or physically handicapped people who are not institutionalized;
- people with mental and psychiatric disorders; and terminal patients who want to die at home.

Some of these groups need home care only for short periods of time, while in other cases, e.g. in chronic disease, it is very difficult to estimate how long home care will be needed. For this (and other) reasons the stress on informal carers differs greatly for different groups of patients.

Interest is growing in early discharge from the hospital and associated home care. For example, early discharge of people after surgery can be a beneficial and cost-effective practice. In the United States, more than 34 percent of all surgical procedures are performed in 'ambulatory surgery' programs, in which people do not remain in the hospital overnight after surgery. Studies show that the outcome in such cases is excellent (75). Providing improved supports in the home could allow more early discharge of people after acute illnesses (10). It is important to realize, though, that people need more education, and probably also need additional home supports, if they are to leave the hospital earlier.

Still, chronic disease (with permanent conditions) is the major issue in home care in the future, especially because of the aging of the population (199;228). Aging is associated with both increases in chronic illness and disability. Overall, about 15 percent of the population of industrialized countries (about 2,2 million people in the Netherlands) have their activities limited by such chronic conditions as heart disease, arthritis and rheumatism, hypertension, and impairments of the back, spine, lower extremities, or hips (186;231). The prevalence of such conditions will probably increase in the future. In the Netherlands, for example, the following trends may be expected, based on extrapolation of recent trends (236):

- an increase in prevalence of many cancers, including cancers of the stomach, lung, breast, ovary, cervix, and prostate (238);
- an increase in accidents;
- an increase in the number of psychosocial problems and a similar prevalence of chronic psychological disorders; and
- an increase in morbidity from chronic degenerative diseases such as respiratory diseases, diabetes, and rheumatoid arthritis.

There is some evidence that aging does not result in an increase in acute care costs per capita. Instead, it results in a significant increase in the intensity of services as functional limitation increases. The most dramatic change is a rise in long-term care expenditures (249).

In the future, the number of disabled will probably increase due not only to the aging of the population. The life expectancy of those with developmental disabilities has increased during the past few decades. Improvements in care for those with traumatic injuries (such as paralysis) have resulted in increased survival and needs for long-term care. Neonatal intensive care is leading to the survival of smaller and smaller infants, and very small infants will probably have an increased prevalence of neurological deficits and other handicapping conditions.

Home care, then, means more than medical services. Many people with functional problems do not need medical services. The condition has been diagnosed. There is no effective cure. Yet the condition causes long-term functional problems. Common performance limitations include (229):

- difficulty in interpreting or processing information;
- severe or complete loss of sight;
- severe or complete loss of hearing;
- poor balance;
- speech or communication problems;
- difficulty in moving the head;
- limitations of stamina or strength;
- difficulty reaching;
- loss of upper extremity skills;
- loss of coordination;
- difficulty handling or fingering (loss of small motor coordination);
- difficulty bending or kneeling;

- reliance on walking aids;
- inability to use the lower extremities.

To stay in the home, many elderly and disabled people need help bathing and in preparing meals. The proportion of those unable to go out of doors and walk down the road unaided increases ten fold between age 65 and age 85 (249).

As will be seen in later sections, many of these problems can be addressed by present or future technology.

Can Home Care Save Resources?

It is often taken for granted that home care can save money for the health care system (26;61;74;201;217;221). It seems apparent that if cheaper home care can substitute for the expensive hospital, money will be saved (119). Likewise, home care makes early discharge from the hospital possible, which is money saving (160).

The evidence as to whether home care does or does not save money is not very extensive, and most of it has been developed in the United States (112). Thus, its applicability to other countries may be limited. Nonetheless, the evidence will be briefly reviewed.

Hedrick and Inui reviewed the evidence for the effectiveness and costs of home care (117). They decided not to include studies that did not meet generally-accepted standards for methodological quality. They were able to identify 12 studies that were either randomized experimental studies or quasi-experimental studies of home care, apparently all conducted in the United States. All programs studied were directed at chronically ill populations. Based on these studies, home care services appear to have no impact on mortality, patient functioning, or nursing home placements (for example, outcomes from home health services were no worse than those from hospital services). Home health services were found either to have no effect on hospitalization or to be associated with an increase in hospital days; ambulatory care utilization was increased as much as 40 percent. Overall costs were either not affected or were increased as much as 15 percent. The authors conclude, " . . . no one should assume that the provision of home care program services will result in diminished utilization of nursing homes, hospitals, or outpatient clinics. . . we are unable to substantiate the contention that home care program services reduce expenditures for medical care." In other words, home health care may result in better care and may meet needs that otherwise would not be met without affecting the overall rate of use of physician and hospital services.

These findings highlight the frequent fear of policy makers that home care services will not result in cost savings because of hidden program costs or potential increase in utilization by people in need who would not otherwise be receiving any services (250).

One important issue concerns the services given by relatives. Ancona-Berk and Chalmers (5) examined the cost of cataract extraction in the hospital compared with ambulatory surgery followed by care in the home. The study was not an experiment, but was based on five simulations of home care. The results indicated that monetary savings were achieved by shortening hospital stays. However, the savings could be attributed to two factors: either fewer services were provided to the home patient or the burden was shifted to relatives.

Zimmer et al (260) studied one sub-population that has been little examined: chronically or terminally ill elderly at high risk of institutionalization. This study was not reported by Hedrick and Inui, probably because it was not published when they completed their work. The study is a randomized controlled study of a home health care team consisting of a physician, nurse practitioner, and medical social worker available, on call, on a 24-hour, seven day per week basis. After randomization, the control group received regular medical services, while the study group received care from the home health care team. The study patients were found to have fewer hospitalizations, nursing home admissions, and outpatient visits than the controls. They were more often able to die at home, if that was their wish. The study group also used more in-home services. The overall costs for the study group were lower than for the controls, but the differences were not statistically significant. The most striking difference was that the patients, and their informal care givers at home, expressed significantly higher satisfaction with the care received than was found in the control group.

One can tentatively conclude, based on these studies, that high quality care can be provided in the home for a number of conditions. Outcomes are generally as good when the care is given at home. Patient satisfaction, as might be expected, is probably higher with home care. However, costs are not significantly lower with expanded home care. Thus, home care seems to be as cost-effective as institutional care, but not necessarily more so. A particularly important issue is that home health care must substitute for other forms of care if it is not to add to costs.

The studies present certain problems in their interpretation. In most of the studies, the patients were not specifically defined. They were chronically-ill people who needed some form of care, not necessarily medical care. This raises the question as to whether specific medical interventions for people traditionally treated in institutions can be delivered in the home at a lower cost.

Even in medical services, the cost of the human element of care is predominant. For example, although the cost of capital and supplies is considerable in providing respiratory care in the home, almost three-quarters of the monthly cost is for nursing care (185, p. 40). (The technologies themselves are described in Section 4.)

One intervention that has been subject to a number of cost-effectiveness analyses is renal dialysis (12;142;157;196). The results of one study will be presented as an example (227). The authors predicted future medical care costs and life expectancy of patient cohorts of 1,000 each in facility dialysis, home dialysis, and cadaveric kidney transplantation over a 10 year period in the United States. The analysis indicated that those in dialysis would have a greater life expectancy than those in the transplant group. The predicted number of years of life was found to be approximately equal for both forms of dialysis, but treatment for the home-dialysis group was found to cost about US$43 million less than for the facility dialysis cohort. The overall costs for home dialysis were found to be 34 percent less than those for facility dialysis.

This issue has also been studied in the Netherlands (48;93). Home dialysis was found to cost about Dfl. 70,000 a year per patient, compared with Dfl. 90,000 for passive center dialysis and Dfl. 80,000 for limited care center dialysis. In 1978 the Health Council stated a quota for home dialysis of 25 percent. Nonetheless, the rate of home dialysis remains low in the Netherlands, about 6 percent in 1985 (159 out of 2,316 patients on dialysis).

Formal cost-effectiveness analyses comparing use of complex technology in home and hospital care have generally not been done, but studies have examined comparative costs between these two sites of care. For example, studies incidate that charges for those requiring ventilator assistance (support for respiration) are approximately 5 to 10 times higher in the hospital than for care in the home. One should note, however, that nursing costs in home care are not included in most of these calculations, nor are the costs of the time of family members (185). Likewise, the differences for the administration of intravenous antibiotics between the two sites are dramatic, in the range of 3-6 to 1. Much more limited evidence also suggests financial savings in cancer chemotherapy and parenteral nutrition (34;69;170; 185;211).

In addition, hospice care has been compared with dying in the hospital. A number of studies on home hospice care claim considerable savings over institutionalized care (24;38;133). Others suggest that there is little or no substitution effect, and that the program may actually increase the total cost of care provided because of the new layer of services added on those already available (45). Coordination of services and re-allocation of funds could solve this problem. In general, home terminal care does improve quality of life at a price that is at least competitive with that of conventional care.

Overall, the available studies of the cost-effectiveness of home care suggest the following conclusions:

1. For chronic illness and functional problems, when continued supportive care is needed, home care is a desirable and effective alternative that can be provided within the limits of present resources. Expectations that developing home care will save money, however, may lead to disappointments.
2. For illness where expensive, high-technology treatments are provided, it may be possible to save societal resources (such as insurance funds), but at least some of the cost will be borne by family and others who provide support in the home.

The studies suggest that careful design of a home care system is essential (58). The goals for such a system must be explicit, so that the system addresses those goals as the most important outcomes.

A Home Care System in Relation to Technology

An innovation is a device, product, or a process introduced to practice for the first time. Technological innovation requires certain conditions. The conditions influencing innovation fall into four categories (181):

- conditions affecting the market for the innovation;
- conditions affecting the ability to appropriate the benefits of the effort to produce the innovation;
- conditions affecting the availability of resources to invest in the innovation; and
- conditions affecting the availability and organization of technical and entrepreneurial know-how.

The market for medical devices for hospital care has been examined and is generally favorable toward innovation in all these respects (181). The result has been very rapid innovation in the hospital sector and intense industrial involvement in this area of innovation. In particular, the market for hospital devices has been largely determined by mechanisms of third party payment (203). The extent of public coverage for hospital care has made the hospital market a stable and rather profitable one.

The hospital system, then, has a number of advantages as a market:

1. the number and types of hospitals are finite and easily identified by industry;
2. the staffs of hospitals include medical specialists who have a great interest in the latest technological innovation; it has been found, for example, that radiologists make up an effective advocate group for new radiological and medical imaging devices within hospitals (104);
3. hospitals have decision-making structures that evaluate innovations and decide whether or not they are worthwhile;
4. hospital devices are publicized and analyzed in lay publications, so that patients often demand them;
5. hospital services are almost entirely covered by public funds or insurance company funds, meaning that patients do not have to worry about the costs of care.

The home health care system, as it exists in most countries today, can hardly be called a system. Services are not entirely covered. They are provided by a number of different agencies and providers in a largely unplanned and uncoordinated fashion. Providers of care in the home are not oriented to modern technology, in general, nor are they trained in the use and maintenance of machines and other devices. The organizations providing home care are also not technologically-oriented.

The Office of Technology Assessment (183), in a report on technology for handicapped people, made the following conclusions:

The disability market population is ill-defined; the economic status of users is often far below the median; disability-related technologies often do not appear salable from a strictly 'market' perspective, resulting in a lack of private interest in their production; product liability is often perceived by manufacturers to be a problem; and especially, the systems for reimbursement of devices sometimes provide disincentives to the marketing of certain types of technologies.

These same generalizations apply to home care in general.

Thus, without changes in the home care system itself, it seems unlikely that new technology will find an important role in home care, nor that industry will find an environment that encourages it to invest in home care technology.

How Can a Home Care System be Developed?

Home care inevitably involves different tasks and different disciplines. No one health care provider can deal with the wide range of medical, social, and functional problems that are presented by those who may need home care. Home care services include, at least, medical services, home nursing, meals on wheels, companions, home makers, home handymen, transportation, and health maintenance services (197). The danger is that the "services a client or patient receives may depend less on assessed needs than on the service array provided by the agency with whom contact is first made" (197).

The key concept is **case management**. Case management means assessing the person's needs and coordinating the activities of professionals and agencies who provide services. The concept is a familiar one in the hospital. The patient's physician is in charge, and orders appropriate diagnostic tests, therapeutic procedures, and nursing care, in consultation with experts in these various other fields. In the home care sector, there is generally no case manager. Who is to be in charge of the assessment process? Who is to have the authority to prescribe needed services? Who is to coordinate different aspects of treatment? Finally, no professional group working in home care at present seems able to take on these tasks. New types of personnel will be needed, or additional training will be needed by present personnel. (The use of the physician as an example is not intended to imply that the case manager in home care should be a physician. The profession chosen may not be the important issue. More important is having the authority. In addition, it is critically important that any group chosen as case managers should be appropriately trained.)

Ultimately, a community and home-centered model of organization of care should involve community access to decision-making and resources. This argument has led some to see home care as primarily a social program rather than a health program (249). The important issue, however, is accountability. In the present situation, no one has the ability to prescribe and coordinate services. This seems to be a necessary condition for developing a true system in home care.

Section 2 – The Present System of Home Care in the Netherlands

The Nature of the Health Care Delivery System

The health care delivery system and policies toward health care delivery are described in more detail in the first report from the project (234), and will only be described briefly here to give a context for home care.

The health care delivery system of the Netherlands is pluralistic. Medical diagnosis and treatment are primarily provided privately. Health care institutions are mostly private, non-profit foundations, although academic and municipal hospitals are public. Doctors and other professionals generally work either in these insitutions or in private practice or in both.

The health care insurance system can be divided into three parts. The first is sick fund insurance, which is a compulsory scheme covering those whose income falls below a certain level. The second part is private insurance, which covers the remaining 40 percent of the population. The third part is General Insurance Against Special Sickness Costs (AWBZ), which covers everyone in the Netherlands for the most expensive forms of care, including long-term care, nursing homes, and mental health services.

Medical specialists are paid fee-for-service for all patients. General practitioners are paid on both a capitation basis and a fee-for-service basis, depending on the patients (general practitioner payment is described in more detail below).

For sick funds or private insurance to pay for specialty or hospital services, a referral by a general practitioner is generally required.

Home Care, Primary Care and First Line Care

This report defines home care by its site: home care is care in the home. This care may be delivered by either professionals or by voluntary care-givers. Thus, it is the site of care that is at the core of the definition. Home care includes medical care, but is broader.

This formulation is not entirely consistent with Dutch policy papers, where the terms 'home care' ('thuiszorg'), 'primary care' and 'first line care' ('eerstelijnszorg') are often used interchangeably. The characteristics of these three forms of care are defined as follows:
- the general character of care
- free access to providers (i.e. without referral)
- situated in the community
- directed towards people in their own environment
- ambulatory care.

The term 'home care' is most related to the third and fourth characteristics. However, this report does not consider that the first two characteristics are essential to home care, for such a definition would exclude specialized home care services such as home dialysis.

The term 'primary care' is usually associated with the general character of care (and possibly the ambulatory character of care). The term 'first line care' refers primarily to free access to the providers; they are the first ones to be consulted in case of health problems and control access to more specialized care.

The defining characteristics indicate that primary care providers such as general practitioners and district nurses have an important role in home care as defined in this report. According to policy papers, this role will increase in the future. Thus, primary care providers are an important group, but the home care system is broader.

Policy Perspectives on Home Care

The Ministry of Welfare, Public Health and Cultural Affairs (WVC), as well as professional organizations, have outlined directions for a home care system in a number of policy papers (162;163;166). Policy towards self care and voluntary care has been stated in a number of governmental notes, including in a note on the rights of patients in general (165), and in a note on care for the elderly in the community

(164). This section will only discuss notes on primary care and home care.

These notes distinguish between three levels of care. The first is the level of informal care: people caring for themselves and for each other (self-care and voluntary care). The second level consists of professional home care and primary care. The third level is made up of specialists and residential care. The core providers of professional home care and primary care are seen as general practitioners, district nurses, family assistants and social workers.

The policy objective outlined in the paper 'Public health in times of restricted finances' (163) is a shift from specialist and residential care to home care and primary care and from professional care to self care and voluntary care. These shifts should be carried out while simultaneously keeping the quality of health care at least at its current level, or even ideally increasing quality.

Key concepts in the 'Note on first line care' (162) are coherence between the three levels of care and tuning to each other of the contributions of the different providers of care at the level of professional home care and primary care. The ideas of coherence and tuning seem to be particular to the organization of health care in the Netherlands as compared to other countries. The policy measures proposed to reach these objectives are known as the 'policy of strengthening primary care.'

Concerning coherence between levels, a number of possible problems can be identified. The possibilities of informal care may be conditional on the supply of services in primary care, for example. Prevention and health education by primary care professionals are essential supporting services. The relation between primary care and specialist and residential care is an important one as a consequence of the strict boundaries between these two levels and the formal requirement of a referral by a general practitioner before a patient may consult with a medical specialist. This requirement applies not only to publicly insured patients; many private insurance carriers also require a letter of referral as a condition for reimbursement.

An important policy objective is to coordinate the supply of professional home care and primary care services. Many of the health-related problems in the population are multi-faceted, with medical, nursing, caring and social aspects. Knowledge of professionals of each others' roles and expertise and cooperation between professionals may make referral or admission to hospital care unnecessary. Research indicates that general practitioners working together in integrated health care centers have lower referral rates, for example (252;253). (It is also important to consider coopration between general practitioners and specialists - this subject will be discussed later.)

Cooperation in professional home care/primary care assumes that different services deal with the same patients. Policy calls for an overlap of catchment populations of the core providers of professional home care/primary care of at least 80 percent. However, catchment areas actually overlap much less. Even in integrated health centers, the rationalization of catchment populations is a problem (30).

The professional organizations of the four core providers of professional home care/primary care have, as a reaction to government policies, united to develop an integrated approach to problems of well-being and health according to a 'general home care concept.' The point of departure is that each profession has its own responsibility and that these responsibilities supplement each other. The providers are to make use of each others' expertise and experience and mutually refer patients and consult each other. At the level of the organization of care, this collaboration should take place for common catchment populations of between 10.000 and 30.000 people. The papers have stated objectives for care given (246):

1. increasing the problem solving capacity of the patient/client;
2. stimulating self care and voluntary care;
3. detecting situations detrimental to health and well being;
4. an integrated psycho-social and medical approach;
5. freedom of the patient/client to decide about the involvement of other professionals;
6. stimulating home care;
7. mutual support of the different professionals.

In conclusion, policies of both government and professional organizations aim at a larger and better organized system of home care and primary care in the Netherlands. Policy measures to reach these aims have been partly successful. The primary care sector has become larger: the list size of general practitioners has decreased considerably (in fact, not as a result of policy measures, but afterwards legitimized by decreases in the normative list size); the volume of subsidies for district nursing has grown; integrated health centers have been subsidized and consequently have grown in numbers.

At the level of organization and coordination, however, policy statements have for the most part remained no more than statements of intention. The actual situation still shows a picture that deviates from the ideals sketched out in the policy notes. Future developments, described in other parts of this report, even point to completely different trends, such as the provision of home care organized by the hospital sector.

Population Groups with Special Needs for Home Care

Although estimates of the size of groups with special needs in the Netherlands could be made, they would be very crude. In addition, they would not take into account the availability of informal care and the specific needs for professional care. Data of this kind can only be collected in studies (e.g. through health interview surveys) designed for this purpose.

In one such study (245), the needs of three groups of patients were surveyed: chronically ill and handicapped people, recently discharged hospital patients, and elderly people with an indication for admission to an old peoples home. The respondents were asked about the kind of care they actually received and the kind of care they felt that they needed. Unmet needs were found first and foremost in the field of assitance in daily living and housekeeping. For each of the three groups, these types of problems were very important, but they were particularly critical for elderly people. For recently discharged patients they were less often the most important.

The 'Core Providers' of Home Care

In policy notes, general practitioners, district nurses, family assistants and general social workers are designated as the 'core providers' of home care. This part describes the situation of each of these professions in Dutch health care (220). Each subpart will have the same structure:

- general information about the number of professionals and their educational background;
- financial arrangements for that group;
- attitudes of those professionals to home care and the relations with other sectors of health care; and

- a description of that part of the work that takes place at the patient's home.

General Practitioners. The medical profession in the home care system is represented by general practitioners. In 1985 there were close to 6000 general practitioners, with an average practice size of about 2450 people (121). Due to the relatively small area of the Netherlands and the high population density, regional disparaties in list size are small. In contrast to more sparcely populated countries, rural areas in the Netherlands are densely doctored, even more so than a lot of urban areas, because general practitioners have extra income opportunities from dispensing pharmaceutical prescriptions and home deliveries (105).

The vocational training of general practitioners consists of a one year post-graduate training program (in existence since 1974); increasing the length of training to two years is being discussed. The program consists of at least six months of residency training with a practising general practitioner, and six months either in general practice or in a general hospital or extended care hospital. During that year students have special courses at the university departments of general practice one day per week. Completion of this training is a condition for an independent general practice.

Nearly all general practitioners are in independent practice; only about 3 percent of them are salaried employees, mainly of foundations that run integrated health centers. The payment system for general practitioners is in part a capitation system and in part a fee-for-service system, depending on the insurance status of the patient. For publicly insured patients (about 62 percent of the population), general practitioners receive a fixed yearly sum (about Dfl. 100,-) directly from the public health insurance funds, irrespective of the services they provide. This sum includes the fee of the general practitioner, a contribution to the cost of pension premiums, and a sum to cover the costs of running the practice, including a salary for a practice assistant or secretary. The actual costs of running the practice are not reimbursed; instead, a lump sum is provided, irrespective of the costs actually incurred. For the other patients (some of whom are not insured for the costs of general practitioner services and some of whom are privately insured), general practitioners are paid on a fee-for-service basis. The system of capitation payments has no incentives to general practitioners to extend home care or to restrict referrals. At the same time, the hospital budget system has changed incentives for the hospital, so hospitals are sending more patients back to general practitioners for their care.

The most common mode of practice is solo practice (59 percent), although the percentage working in solo practice has been declining steadily during the past ten years, falling from 75 percent in 1975 (121).

Little research into the attitudes of general practitioners towards home care has been done. Related research has been done, however, covering such topics as the demarcation of the tasks of specialists and general practitioners, referrals, psychosocial aspects of complaints of patients, preventive care, and terminal care. Attitudes of general practitioners vary quite a lot, but a few indications of their attitudes can be presented.

As far as the demarcation of tasks of medical specialists and general practitioners is concerned, research shows (17;18;204;205;206;207; 208;239) that general practitioners generally carry out more tasks than medical specialists consider desirable or justified. Research into the determinants of the referral rate of general practitioners (63) indicates that general practitioners who see more illnesses as belonging to their field of competence, who have critical attitudes towards specialist care, and who provide more therapeutic interventions (mainly in the field of minor surgery), tend to have lower referral rates. Psychosocial backgrounds or aspects of complaints of patients are more readily recognized and treated by general practitioners with a more general medical orientation as compared to those with a more technical somatic orientation, and by general practitioners who consider the treatment of psychosocial complaints as an integral aspect of their work (244).

The working style of general practitioners seems to be at odds with the requirements of active screening and prevention (33; 193;194; 198). Less than half of Dutch general practitioners consider periodic screening of high risk groups to be part of their task (111). This may be indicative of an unfavourable attitude towards preventive care, but it could also reflect a critical attitude towards the value of active screening.

Terminal care is nearly unanimously accepted as an important task of general practitioners, but of course the amount of terminal care needed depends heavily on the number of patients dying at home. In

1980 approximately 40 percent of deaths occurred at home (47), but of course not all people dying at home need terminal care. On the other hand, some people have terminal care, but finally die in hospital.

The clearest indicator of the role of the general practitioner in home care is the extent of home visits. No data are available on this subject, but only estimates. It is estimated that one in five consultations is a home visit (118, p.17). In rural areas home visits are more usual than in urban areas. In the past decade the number of home visits seems to have declined (219).

Exact data on the content of home care is not available. Nor is it known for what group of patients and for what kind of complaints home visits are made. It is not known what kind of services are given. The lack of data on the amount and kind of services of general practitioners is a general problem of Dutch general practice, related to the system of payment (88). A national study of morbidity and interventions in general practice is presently being carried out by NIVEL.

District Nurses. In contrast to general practitioners, district nurses are not in independent practice, but are employed by the so-called cross-organizations (Kruis-organisaties). Cross-work is organized at different levels. The organizational structure is given in figure 1.

```
                  National Cross-organization
                              |
                              |
                              |
                          Head units  (mainly at the provincial
                              |         level)
                              |
                              |
                              |
                 Regional Cross-organizations
                              |
                              |
                              |
                        Basic teams  (Local Cross-organizations)
```

Figure 1 Organizational structure of the Cross-work Organizations

Employment for district nurses is with the more than 200 regional cross-organizations. These regional organizations are made up of a number of basic teams, typically consisting of a head nurse, seven registered nurses and two unregistered nurses (called 'ziekenverzorgenden'). The total number of head nurses, registered nurses, and unregistered nurses is estimated to be about 5,900. The number of people per registered nurse is about 3,000. The education of registered district nurses is either the normal education of hospital nursing, followed by a two year course in public health, or the four year higher vocational training in nursing.

Since 1980, the services of district nurses have been financed through a system of public insurance (for the whole of the Dutch population), based on the General Insurance Against Special Sickness Costs (AWBZ). To actually use the services of district nurses one has to be (or become) a member of the local cross-organization. The membership fee may be considered as a kind of copayment.

The services of district nurses are directly accessable to the population, that is to say: people may use the services without referral by a physician.

There seems to be a discrepancy between what district nurses consider important tasks and the expectations of patients and of other health care professionals (137). While patients and other professionals expect district nurses to provide nursing services, district nurses themselves consider support and psychosocial care as an increasingly important task. In fact, hospital nursing and district nursing show opposite trends in their development in this respect during the past decade. Hospital nursing is characterized by increasing specialization, rationalization, and use of machine technology. District nursing, however, emphasizes all-round nursing, attention to psychosocial aspects of people's problems, and a supportive attitude. While these are beneficial services, there is an impression growing that bedside nursing tends to be neglected. This is an important issue if home care is to be an alternative to institutional care.

Most of the work of district nurses is home care in the strict sense of the word, with the exception of well-baby care, which in part takes place at the office of the local cross-organization. It is estimated (174) that approximately 9 percent of the Dutch population receives care of district nurses. Of course, the percentage of the population in care of district nurses varies with age (see Table 1). The kinds of services provided by district nurses also vary with the age of the patients (Table 2).

Table 1 Percentage of the population by age group cared for by district nurses

age group	percentage in care
0- 4	72,5 %
5-14	1,3 %
15-19	0,4 %
20-39	2,6 %
40-59	2,0 %
60-69	7,3 %
70-79	24,2 %
80	59,4 %

Source: 174, table 6.

Note: The high percentage in the 0 to 4 years of age group is due to the fact that well baby care is organized as part of the work of district nurses in the Netherlands.

Overall, the most important group of services concern the field of physical care and personal hygiene. Health education is the second most common service, followed by administration of medicine and nursing services, such as injections and care of wounds. Health education is more common in the younger age groups, because of well baby care and pre- and postnatal care (age group of 20-39 years). The categories of services reported by the cross-organizations are rather broad; it is therefore not possible to determine how much of the work of district nurses is in care for the dying, for example.

Two special (and important) topics in district nursing will be discussed later; these are the continuous availability (day and night and during week-ends) of nursing services and the organization of post-hospitalization home care.

The Social Work System. There are approximately 180 more-or-less regionalized institutions of social work. These institutions are independent foundations employing altogether about 2,300 general social workers. The social work system is mainly financed through governmental subsidies (about 85 percent Rijksbijdrageregeling) and

Table 2 Kind of services provided by district nurses by age of the patient as a percentage of the number of contacts (excluding well baby care consultation at the office of the local cross-organization).

kind of service	0-1	1-4	5-14	15-19	20-39	40-59	60-69	70-79	80+	Total (%)
- intake	0.7	1.7	2.0	2.2	2.3	1.8	1.5	1.4	1.0	1.2
- physical care and hygiene	0.6	1.2	7.4	19.5	18.7	36.2	37.3	36.7	49.0	33.0
- nursing services	2.5	0.6	2.7	31.1	9.5	20.1	17.9	18.6	16.7	16.0
- administration of medicines	0.2	0.1	3.6	6.0	3.6	15.9	22.3	23.5	20.1	18.0
- reactivation	-	0.1	0.8	0.6	2.1	1.8	1.9	1.9	1.6	1.0
- support in realizing therapy or regimen	1.5	1.0	12.1	8.5	7.4	8.1	6.3	5.9	3.9	4.8
- support in problem situations	1.4	2.2	15.4	8.8	16.4	11.4	8.0	4.9	3.5	5.1
- health education	82.2	87.0	55.3	23.1	39.9	4.7	5.2	7.1	4.2	20.1
- screening	10.9	6.1	0.7	0.2	0.1	0	0	0	0	0.8
total										100%

Source: 174, tables 7 and 8

in part through municipal and other subsidies. In the larger cities both the social work system and family assistants are financed by the municipalities.

The education of social workers is a four year higher vocational training, including one year of practical work. There is a possibility of continued education during two years on a part-time basis.

The services of general social workers are directly accessible to the population and free of charge.

Part of social work is done in collaboration with primary health care professionals (general practitioners and district nurses) through participation in integrated health centers or so-called 'home teams.' The goal of this collaboration is to coordinate the services of different professionals. Many complaints of patients to general practitioners or district nurses have social or psychological aspects. Cooperation of social workers with these professionals should prevent extended medical treatment of people with essentially psychosocial complaints.

Many social workers, however, reject close cooperation with health professionals, because they fear a 'medicalization' of social problems (138).

For a few specific aspects of social work related to health care, research has been done on the opinions of social workers (29;31). Social workers in integrated health centers are involved in care for the dying and support in mourning. This last aspect is quantitatively more important in their work and social workers are more satisfied with their role in giving support during mourning than with their tasks in care for the dying. Social workers have a positive attitude towards collective and individual aspects of prevention of psychosocial problems.

The organization of social work institutions ('JOINT') distinguishes the following tasks of social workers (see the review by Kersten) (139):

- counseling (support of people with psycho-social problems and intervention in crisis situations)
- information and advice
- mediation between the client and care organizations
- referral of clients to other professionals
- handling things on behalf of the client, such as writing of appeals detection of societal problems
- stimulating and supporting self care
- support of voluntary workers.

Counseling is the most important kind of service (nearly half of the clients receive counseling).

It is estimated that approximately 2,4 percent of the Dutch population is in contact with the social work system. In many cases, people contact a general social worker on advice of their general practitioner. Data on the extent of home care by social workers, in the sense of consultations in the client's home, is not available.

Family Assistants. Family assistance aims to help in households where the normal way of living is disturbed, because one of the members of the household is not able to carry burdens due to illness or disability.

There are approximately 240 local or regional institutions of family assistance (in a number of cases combined with the institutions of general social work) employing about 30,000 family assistants (in full-time equivalents) and another 18,000 on a kind of free lance basis, mediated by the institutions. The number of employees has decreased during the past decade, while there is a growing share of free lance workers in family assistance. Institutions of family assistance are financed through subsidies from the national government (Ministry of Welfare, Public Health and Cultural Affairs).

The education of family assistants is generally lower vocational training, but there is a differentiation according to education and experience. Family assistants are allocated to households according to their level of education and experience and the needs of the household.

The tasks of family assistance are housekeeping (which is quantitatively the most important task), personal care, and (social) support. The number of clients receiving family assistance was about 185,000 in 1984, mainly elderly people (72 percent) and chronically ill people (13 percent). Clients of family assistance get an average of 12 hours of help per week (see the review by Boerma) (28).

Eligibility for family assistance is based on uniform rules and criteria (not always uniformly applied). Every six months a re-assessment of the clients is required to assure that the assistance given still meets the needs of the client.

Eligibility is based on questions such as these:
- is assistance necessary or is voluntary care available?
- is family assistance necessary or are there alternative facilities?
- what kind of assistance is necessary, what level of education or experience should the assistant have?
- what is the expected duration of assistance?
- how urgent is the request compared to other requests?

Requests for family assistance are made either by the clients themselves (one third of the elderly clients and two thirds of the other clients) or through mediation of the general practitioner, district nurse, or social worker.

Clients must pay part of the costs of family assistance themselves. The amount of copayment is based on the financial resources of the household. The average amount of copayment has increased during the past decade.

Integrated Provision of Home Care Services

The 'core providers' of home care each work in different circumstances. The financing of their services differs, the way they are paid differs, and the way that patients or clients enter the system differs. These differences have impeded the working together of those providers.

One attempt to deal with this problem has been the development of health centers in which professionals of different kinds work together. (The Almere project, another approach, is described later in this section.) The number of integrated health centers does not exceed 150. By definition, general practitioners, district nurses, and social workers practice in all of these centers, but family assistance is involved in only 20 percent of the health centers. Only 7 percent of general practitioners work in health centers. The centers have an average of 3 general practitioners, 3 district nurses, and one and a half social workers.

The philosophy behind health centers is that many patient complaints are not simply medical problems, but have a social or psychological background or need nursing care. The treatment of these complaints might be better when general practitioners, social workers, and district nurses discuss patient problems, consult each other when necessary, refer to each other, or treat patients together. Specifically, from the point of view of home care, it could be argued that patients who need home care in most cases need different kinds of care (e.g., medical care and nursing care). The coordination of care provided by different professionals to the same patient might be easier when the professionals involved work together in a health center.

Whether this philosophy is indeed actually implemented in integrated health centers is difficult to say. Results of research in one field - that of referrals from general practitioners to medical specialists - are positive. General practitioners in health centers have lower numbers of referrals to medical specialists.

In addition to integrated health centers, there are looser forms of cooperation in the form of home teams. In home teams, the core providers of home care cooperate without sharing the same premises. At the moment, there are more than 400 home teams. It is important to note that family assistance services more often participate in home teams than in integrated health centers.

One problem in developing closer cooperation between the different core providers is the lack of knowledge of how they actually spend their time and what expertise each has. Developing an arbitrary system for coordination of services is likely to fail for this reason. Any move toward developing structures for coordination and communication must be done carefully, with full involvement of those involved in home care.

Some Special Topics in Home Care

A number of problems in the Dutch system of home care may be identified. The last part of this Section is devoted to a discussion of these problems.

In a health care system with clear boundaries between first line or primary health care and other sectors of health care, there may be problems when people move from one sector to another. Two topics related to this problem will be discussed here: the field of rehabilitation and discharge from the hospital.

Home Care and Rehabilitation. The 'core providers' of home care form - at least to some extent - a system of health care. Providers of care in the field of rehabilitation are organized apart from this. However, the field of rehabilitation, aids, and adaptations for the disabled is an important dimension of home care.

The ultimate goal of rehabilitation is to help disabled people to get or keep a place in society suited to their potentialities. A goal for the system is to keep full admissions to rehabilitation centers as short as possible (or, ideally, to prevent them altogether).

There are about 1,900 beds in rehabilitation clinics, 8 ambulatory rehabilitation centers, and a number of day care rehabilitation departments of general hospitals. In the case of rehabilitation, the same kind of policy as described earlier is advocated: a shift from clinical treatment to day care treatment to ambulatory treatment to home care. These shifts imply an increasing share of self care and home care, either by professionals or by the informal social network (243). As far as professionals are involved, there are two possibilities: first, members of the rehabilitation team can step outside the clinic and treat and care for patients at home; second, the rehabilitation team can transfer the treatment and/or care to other professionals such as general practitioners, district nurses, or physiotherapists. As far as the first possibility is concerned, some experiments are being conducted. The main problem with this option is that the typical approach of rehabilitation, that is, a multidisciplinary treatment by a team of professionals, is difficult to realize in the patient's home. It is possible for individual team members to treat patients at home, but this does not seem to be efficient when a whole team has to visit a patient. Furthermore, the equipment of rehabilitation centers facilitates treatment. There must then be a careful selection of patients and/or stages in the rehabilitation process to make treatment and care at home feasible.

For the second possibility, it is important to note that from the point of view of the rehabilitation team there may be doubts about the skills of general practitioners, district nurses and private physiotherapists in taking over the treatment of patients. The minimum for post-clinic patients is communication between the rehabilitation team and primary health care (as individual professionals or as a team) to transfer treatment and care. If a multidisciplinary approach continues to be necessary, someone must take responsibility for coordinating the home care/treatment. Recent research indicates that there is not much communication in this respect (254). The uneven spatial distribution of rehabilitation facilities may be a structural restriction to arranging outreach and transfer of treatment by rehabilitation teams.

The transfer of treatment and care from rehabilitation teams to primary health care may have its problems, but the possibilities of primary health care must not be underestimated. In the foregoing sections, the work of general practitioners, district nurses, social workers and family assistants has been discussed. District nurses, especially, have a task in reactivating patients, give assistance in daily living (ADL) training, and so on. Apart from these 'core providers' of home care, there is a large number of physiotherapists in the Netherlands (approximately 12,000). At least two thirds of them work outside the clinical setting in private practices. It may be questioned to what extent their work can be labelled as 'rehabilitation.' It lacks the multidisciplinary team approach and the explicit orientation towards social integration. Still, for disabled people and chronically ill and elderly patients, physiotherapy aims at keeping them in the community and preventing admission to nursing homes. Although most of the treatments by private physiotherapists take place at physiotherapy practices, 15 percent of treatments take place at the patient's home. This percentage is considerably larger in the case of chronically ill patients: approximately 40 percent, and for some categories of patients it is even higher, e.g., for patients with diseases of the respiratory system (106).

Home care for handicapped people largely depends on the possibilities to secure aids and adaptations of the living environment of patients. The provision of aids and adaptations is regulated in a number of social security acts and regulations, the most important of which are the General Disability Act, the Health Insurance Fund Act, and the General Act on Exceptional Medical Expenses. The main advisory institution on requests for aids and adaptations for people below the age of 65 years is the Gemeenschappelijke Medische Dienst (89). The annual reports of this institution give insights in the kind of aids and adaptations that are provided. The biggest category is adaptations of the house (and within this category adaptation of the bathroom); the second biggest category is provision for mobility outside the house (mainly compensation for transport costs); the third biggest is aids for ADL (assistance in daily living).

Problems in this field are that there are a number of different acts, each with its own conditions and regulations, while people may have difficulties in finding the right channel for their problems. In addition, it takes time for request, assessment, advice, and provision of a solution. For short term problems, e.g., in post-hospitalization home care, the course of providing services is not adequate.

Some devices are available from the loan desk of the district nursing organizations (the Cross-work organization).[2] The number and scope of aids available differs from region to region. The regional organizations are autonomous on matters such as purchase, maintenance, and distribution of aids, while the National Cross-organization plays mainly an advisory role. The policy is to let the specific needs in the area involved determine the availability of aids. In practice, most devices are bought through the National Cross-organization, and its guidelines for inventory lists are used as a starting point. The inventory list includes about 50 items, mostly rather low technology in nature, such as devices to raise and lower beds, devices dealing with bathing and using the toilet, and containers for urine and sputum. A few more sophisticated aids, such as anti-decubitus mattresses and wheelchairs, are available at a more centralized level.

Organization of Post-hospitalization Home Care. One of the groups with special needs for home care is made up of people who are recently discharged from the hospital, although, of course, not all patients discharged from the hospital need after-care. What makes this group particularly interesting is the fact that at discharge from the hospital patients are transferred from one sector of the health care system - the hospital sector - to another one - primary health care or the informal care of relatives and neighbours. As a result of the rather strict boundaries between sectors of health care in the Dutch system, the transfer from one sector to another may give problems in the coordination of care. For example, general practitioners need to be informed when a patient on their list is discharged, but if this happens at all, it is often very late, due to administrative delays.

Coordination is generally seen as a task for nursing. Organizationally, this has been dealt with by creating a new function: the nurse in charge of the continuity of care of discharged patients (144). The flow of information is regulated through the use of specially designed transfer forms which are filled in by the hospital nurses or the special nurse and are sent to the district nurse. The nurse charged with the continuity of care may be involved in the selection of hospital patients who are expected to need extra

---

[2]) Information in this paragraph was acquired by a staff member of TNO, who visited the National Cross-organization and two local Cross-work organizations on behalf of the project. He commented that present maintenace is well-carried out, but that the organizations were not prepared to assess or maintain more sophisticated devices.

(nursing) care after discharge, in notifying the district nurse that the patient is going to be discharged, and generally in coordinating, stimulating and supporting the cooperation between hospital and district nursing. There are some twenty nurses specially charged with the continuity of care of discharged patients. They work only in parts of the country; in other parts the transfer of information on patients to be discharged is directly from the hospital to the district nursing organization.

Based on case studies, it is estimated that approximately 10 percent of discharged patients receive home care after discharge (that is, 150,000 patients). Some groups of patients are more likely to receive professional home care then others: young children, elderly people, women, and people without access to informal care. Home care is mainly given after major surgery or after long hospitalization for chronic diseases.

Substitution, in the sense of shorter length of stay in the hospital in combination with organized home care after discharge, has not generally been demonstrated to occur. There has been little research into the merits of different ways of organizing and coordinating home care after discharge from the hospital. However, the projects to be described next are surely resulting in a shorter length of stay in hospital overall.

Home Care by Hospital-Based Specialists. The appropriateness of home care for some medical conditions, especially with technological advances, and the lack of alternative provisions for medical care in the home has led to some attempts by hospital-based specialists to provide home care. In some cases, the care given is too specialized in any case to be provided by a general practitioner. Theoretically, any hospital specialist in the Netherlands could be involved in home care. For example, the resuscitation department of the University of Utrecht provides respiratory care in the home. This part, then, is not intended to be complete.

The Free University of Amsterdam began a project to improve cooperation between primary care providers and specialists in 1985. The general objective is to care for the patient at the level and site best suited to the problem. Thus, the project includes specialists involved in home care and general practitioners involved in hospital care. A steering committee made up of primary care providers and hospital staff considers proposed projects and selects those that seem feasible. Projects underway include treatment of respiratory problems in children, treatment of type 2 diabetes mellitus, ambulatory surgery (without hospital admission), diet management in mild to moderate hypertension, and care for open leg ulcers. Other projects have been suggested or approved, including cancer therapy, treatment of hypertension, treatment of dietary allergy in infants, treatment of sports injuries, and provision of advice on genetic problems. In the ambulatory surgery project, for example, the general practitioner is involved in planning the surgery. Procedures being done in the project include repair of inguinal hernia, repair of varicose veins, removal of synthetic materials from bone after healing, and removal of benign lesions such as tumors. The patient returns home after the condition is stable, and the general practitioner supervises subsequent care, with the assistance of a district nurse, if necessary. Outcomes of these projects are being evaluated, with emphasis on both costs of care and quality of life for the patients. The overall project is considered to use a method widely applicable in the Netherlands.

Continuous Accessability of Home Nursing Services, Family Assistance, and General Social Work. Another potential set of problems is the different status of the professions involved in home care. General practitioners are mainly self-employed, while the other professionals are employees of larger organizations. The need for home care does not stop at the closing of office hours. In fact, only general practitioners are continuously accessible, either personally or through a system of deputies. However, during the last few years experiments have been done in continuous accessibility of district nursing, family assistance, and general social work, and some localities have now made such accessibility a part of their systems. The introduction of continuous accessibility in these other areas is furthest advanced in district nursing, followed by the social work institutions. Family assistance is still far from ideal in this regard.

The availability of professional care in evenings, nights and weekends serves the following functions:

- caring for patients whose situation demands one or more visits, not only during the day but also outside office hours;
- taking the pressure off informal carers;
- giving the patient and informal carers the feeling of security that they can always rely on professional care.

The introduction of continuous nursing care in the home situation has been accompanied by evaluation research in a number of cases (23;149).

Most of the people who use the services of district nurses in the evening and at night are elderly people (three quarters of the users) who are not living alone. The availability of informal care is seen as important for the coordination of care.

The patients are either chronically ill or terminal patients. The most common diagnoses are cancers and diseases of the circulatory system. As in district nursing in general, in the evening and at night, the biggest part of care is consumed by a small number of patients who need care for a long period of time (chronically ill patients). The number of persons recently discharged from the hospital is relatively small in the group of patients who receive evening and night home nursing care.

Continuous home nursing services are therefore important as a substitute for admissions to nursing homes (at least in the perception of district nurses themselves), but are of minor importance for shortening the length of stay in hospitals up to the present. However, since continuous nursing is generally not available, patients are kept in hospital until their conditions are well-stabilized and a minimum of care is necessary. Shortening length of stay in hospital would seem to require greater availability of home nursing services.

There have been no extensive cost-benefit studies of continuous home nursing services, but Besteman et al (23) indicate that the costs of evening and night home nursing are less than the costs of admission to a nursing home or general hospital.

Van Sonderen (222) reported on the evaluation of an experiment in family assistance. The experiment aimed at:

- making care directly available (without a waiting list);
- promoting continuity of care;
- making care flexible, that is, adapted to the needs and wishes of the clients;
- stimulating and supporting self-care and informal care.

It was hoped that this orientation by family assistants would prevent or delay admission to a hospital or nursing home and would shorten the stay of admitted patients. Van Landern concluded that admissions were prevented or delayed in a number of cases, but that the length of stay was not shorter in cases where continuous assistance was possible.

An important organizational problem is how to phase-out and eventually stop the care at home. Since budgets are restricted, services need to be stopped as soon as possible to enable the services to take on new clients. This is an unsolved problem in these services.

The Almere Health Care Project. The Almere health care project was established in 1983 as an experiment with the aim of strengthening primary health care and supported by the Ministry of Welfare, Public Health, and Cultural Affairs (WVC). The project is organized through health centers that employ all health care workers. At the same time, the project includes consultation and cooperation with other care givers, including nursing homes, hospitals, and mental health institutions. The aim is to develop care to meet certain needs, especially those of the elderly. An important part of the project is developing means of improved information flow between providers.

The cooperating organizations have formed a local health care body that makes a year joint health care budget. Part of the budget includes special funds to support home care in Almere. These special funds have been obtained by reducing the planned hospital by 60 beds.

The aim of the project is a coherent and humane structure for health care at a reasonable cost. Such a structure should be more receptive to advanced technology in the home. Extensive evaluations are being carried out. It is hoped that the project will have important results and will provide a model for the future of home care in the Netherlands.

Problems of the Home Care Sector: Is It Yet a System?

The most important criticism of the home care system of the Netherlands is that it hardly merits the term 'system.' Providers deliver home care services. People receive services in their homes. Resources are invested in home care. Home care services are based on or provide technologies. However, these services and people are not related to each other in a planned, coordinated system.

Problems at the Policy Level. As the review of policy papers on home care showed, the definition of home care is not clear. Home care is equated with first line or primary health care, but in a logical definition, it should at the same time be smaller (only care given at the patient's home) and broader (also including specialist care given at home). Due to this lack of a clear definition, there is no attention to the growing role of hospitals or other institutions such as rehabilitation centers in home care.

Ideally, the goal for home care services is to promote autonomy of the person receiving the service. A subsidiary goal might be to be certain that those who provide the bulk of home care families, neighbors, and friends are given effective support from an organized services system.

General Criticisms of Home Care. Multiple organizations are involved in home care, each with its own priorities, methods of collecting its resources, methods of paying its staff, and methods of determining who needs its services. In addition, general practitioners are usually private physicians in solo or group practice. The organizations have different and sometimes overlapping catchment areas, so that it may be difficult or even impossible for a particular patient to receive coordinated services, even with the best will of the providers.

At the level of day to day care there are problems in the coordination of services. Within primary health care there is the problem that all professions involved have their own organization and statute. Coordination of the services through integrated health centers is quantitatively of minor importance at present. Whenever the care crosses the boundaries between sectors in the health care system, problems of coordination arise. In post-hospitalization home care, an organizational solution is sought in the creation of a special function, that of the nurse in charge of the continuity of care for discharged patients. An important question is who is to coordinate home care (if the patient and his informal carers cannot take this responsibility any more). The answer to this question will shape the future of home care.

Communication between the different providers and provider organizations is minimal. Each organization tends to make its own decision as to whether a person needs their services or not. There is no common standard for defining needs, and there is no one doing a needs assessment and prescribing services to meet those needs.

For medical functions, a GP wishing to provide diagnostic or therapeutic services in either clinic or home needs good back-up by more specialized personnel, including especially the chance to consult on problems, without being required to actually refer the patient. These opportunities are mostly lacking in the Netherlands.

In summary, although the Netherlands invests considerably in home care, the investment is uncoordinated and is in no way clearly connected to community needs.

Problems in Financing Home Care Services. The pluralism of the health care system of the Netherlands is perhaps nowhere more apparent than in the field of home care. Multiple organizations pay for home care. Again, these different payment sources are in no way coordinated. There are important gaps in people's coverage for home care, and also multiple overlaps. It is worth noting that insurance companies in the Netherlands have begun to pay for home care, including home nursing, as an alternative to institutional care.

A very visible problem in home care is the differing methods of paying practitioners. This is perhaps more visible in home care because a high percentage, perhaps 80 percent of resources, go for salaries. Payment of general practitioners, who are paid by capitation, is a particular problem in attempts to encourage home care. Capitation is a system of payment with an incentive for delivering fewer services. The general practitioner actually loses resources every time he or she provides services. The incentive in this system is to refer any patient needing diagnostic, therapeutic, or rehabilitative services to a specialist. The specialist is willing to take the referral, because providing the service adds to his or her income.

With this payment system, it seems unlikely that GPs can accept an expanded role in providing or supporting home care services.

The insurance system has other problems. Many people are privately insured for specialist and hospital care, but not for GP care. The people would obviously prefer immediate referral to a specialist, where their services are covered.
Another problem concerns levels of payment. These are low, especially for family assistants, who have little specific training. Home care in general is not a prestigious field. Improving home care seems to require improved payment levels for staff, but this also implies the

higher prestige that would go with more formal training programs. Thus, payment, education, and prestige are intertwined.

The fragmentation of the payment system goes hand-in-hand with the lack of a system.

Problems in the Personnel of Home Care. Designing a future system of home care requires thinking in terms of functions to be fullfilled and not (only) in terms of manpower. The process of aging of the population does not necessarily require an equivalent growth in the number of, e.g., district nurses. It may require certain functions already more than amply available as well as new functions.

Home care providers, including GPs, nurses, and social workers are all quite psychosocial in their orientation. This orientation should not be lost. However, technical skills of physicians and nurses are not well-developed. Delivering medical care at home requires that the GP be better trained and supported in this area. The same is true of nurses.

Because of this lack, at least in part, some hospital specialists are moving into home care in some instances. At present, there are few opportunities for specialists and generalists to interact in constructive ways. There is a need for models of cooperation between such providers.

In summary, what is needed is a careful assessment of future needs, followed by appropriate training programs to assure that individuals are available with the necessary skills.

Problems with Technology in Home Care. The problems in providing technology, especially medical technology, in home care are multiple. It is not clear who should prescribe the technology who is to do the needs assessment and match a technology to the needs? Providers are not trained to select technologies for home care, nor are they trained in the use of technologies in the home. They may not have a positive attitude toward technology in the home.

In the case of complicated technologies, especially machines, there is no clear system for maintenance, and the back-up for those providing care in the home is not clear. Patients may be afraid of equipment failures or other emergencies; without a good system for dealing with such problems, people will probably not accept home care for medical conditions.

In some cases, systems have developed. For patients with insulin pumps, a specialist is available in the hospital on a 24-hour basis. Some industrial suppliers also offer round-the-clock service.

The payment system often does not cover technology in the home, or covers it only partially. If the technology is part of specialty medical care, it probably is covered. For example, home dialysis is fully covered by the Sick Funds (93, pp. 150-156). The situation with aids is not so clear, however. There are many sources of payment, including Sick Funds, disability laws, pension funds, and general insurance against special sickness (AWBZ). Devices for assistance in daily living (ADL), for example, is covered by all sources of funds (126). Other specific aids may not be paid for by any source. It is difficult for the individual to know where to seek help.

Equipment used in home care functions with limited professional supervision, which means that problems cannot be detected and addressed immediately. This indicates that special attention needs to be paid to construction of such equipment. Reliability should have the highest priority for equipment intended for use in the home.

A final problem is that there are few provisions for teaching people (patients) and families how to use technology in the home.

Problems for the Patient in Home Care. The main problems for the patient in home care are apparent from the foregoing discussion. The patient does not have a clear entry point for home care. Should he or she go to a general practitioner? Or approach a Cross-work Organization? Or contact the social work institution? What are the advantages and disadvantages of each of these routes? Who is to decide which patients can gain the most from home care?

For the patient, the critical issue concerning home care and technology used in the home is that it be well-suited to his or her needs. This requires a careful diagnosis and needs assessment, followed by a prescription. Who is to carry out this task? And how are physical, psychic, and social aspects of a patient's problems to be dealt with in an integrated way?

For planning a home care system, data is needed on patient needs. However, little is known about such needs. The hospital system produces copious data on the nature and types of services provided. No such data is produced by the home care sector.

Finally, the patient will find few opportunities to learn to use technology in the home.

An important and increasing role is played by patient organizations, which both act politically and provide direct help to people with certain diseases or conditions. For example, organizations have grown up around such problems as multiple sclerosis, cancer, congenital genetic diseases, and cardiovascular disease. Information concerning these conditions and possible treatment or assistance is available through these organizations.

Conclusions

The home care system in the Netherlands is not well-developed. The best part of the system is that it does have resources and services are being provided to people. The worst part is that no one knows if these are appropriate services, much less if they are the most appropriate services.

A true system requires planning for the intelligent use of available resources. It requires coordination between those resources. And it requires evaluation to see how well the job has been done and to change how it will be done in the future. These elements are critically lacking in the Netherlands.

This Section has focused on those providing home care. Of course, these 'core providers' are not the only ones involved in such care. One should also be aware of others who may provide care to people remaining in the home, including occupational and physical therapists, speech therapists, pharmacists, and hospital specialists (130;230).

The policy conclusions presented in Section 7 are intended to begin to address these problems. An important policy report completed in 1987 by a Commission chaired by Professor Dekker made recommendations addressed to some of the problems identified in this Section (50). In particular, the Commission pointed out the problems in the financing systems, specifying both the different system for different practitioners and the capitation payment system for general practitioners as problems. The Commission supported the strengthening of primary care and home care because of cost-effectiveness considerations. The report has been transmitted to the government and seems likely to lead to significant changes in the system described in this Section.

Part II – General Introduction to Technologies for Home Care

Industrialized societies are experiencing an ongoing technological revolution that started some two decades ago. As a result new technological developments are expected to transform homes, affecting the nature and potential of home care services in the future. For example, industry expects the home care market for equipment and supplies to grow at the rate of 20 to 25 percent annually (155).

In the following sections of this report, a wide range of future developments in home care technology will be discussed. The definition of technology used in this report is broad, including not only devices, drugs, and procedures, but also the organizational and supportive systems within which care is provided. For this reason, the first section following this introduction deals with some possible future changes in home care technology that do not involve physical artefacts.

The subsequent sections deal primarily with artefacts. The first of these sections focuses on traditional clinical or medical technologies, which at present are rapidly moving into the home and make home care an alternative to hospital care in many instances. The second section deals with those future advances in technology that are addressed to enhancing functioning of those with chronic conditions in the home, thereby increasing the possibility of independent living for these individuals. The last section is directed towards advances in information technology, an area of very rapid technological change.

A number of areas of technological change that are of importance to future home care were excluded from this report: architecture and urban planning, transportation, and working in the home, for example.

Technological innovations in the home raise some basic issues. The first issue concerns human care versus machine-based care in the home care system of the future. Historically, home care services have been people- or labor-intensive. In the coming years, many of the functions of human care can be supported by machine-based technology, or even taken over by machines. A central question for the future is this: which tasks will be performed by machines, and which tasks will be kept within the domain of people? Clearly, the application of future home care devices opens up many new possibilities, both for the individual him or herself and for the caregiver. If, however, these artefacts are to contribute to cost-effective and high quality home care and self-care, their capabilities and limits need to be understood. Furthermore, in an environment of accelerating technological change, alternative and competing technologies will emerge to address the same problem. Thus, it is not sufficient to examine specific technologies. Analyses must compare the costs and benefits of various care systems, including technological options that exist and emerge. These comparisons should not be based only on efficiency and cost-effectiveness issues, but also must take into account how the various technological options can contribute to 'humane' care and quality of life. Home care has always been oriented to care of people. This valuable orientation must not be lost through the spread of complex technology into the home.

A second issue which merits specific attention concerns the man-machine interface. While the technical possibilities in home care are manifold, the usefulness of these tools - which will often be used by elderly people or those with chronic handicapping conditions - depends heavily on their 'user-friendliness.' New technologies are often not very well adapted to the (technological) capability of the user. Devices could be designed so they are much easier to use. For example, microprocessors are becoming universal in home appliances and do not necessarily require training for their use. At the same time, one should remember that attitudes toward technology will change. Today's middle-aged people are tomorrow's elderly. Whereas today elderly people are often not familiar with advances in such fields as computers, tomorrow's elderly people will be quite different in many respects. In summary, much more work is needed on the issue of man-machine interface.

A third issue concerns devices for functioning. Devices to assist handicapped people have received a great deal of attention. Devices for elderly people, in contrast, have received little specific attention. Available devices are usually addressed to a specific disease or disability. Devices to assist in problems of everyday living are much harder to identify.

The fourth issue focuses on the fact that one of the advantages of home care is that it can be provided in the individual's own home environment and not in an institutional setting. Thus, when considering technological solutions and their industrial design, one must be careful not to transfer an institutional atmosphere into the home. In many situations, it may be most desirable to modify or adapt existing furniture or household items rather than introducing new equipment. A simple example can illustrate the point. Present-day faucets (taps) in the home are often operated by turning knobs, which is a problem for those with rheumatism and arthritis. In contrast, taps used in laboratories can be operating by using elbows and underarms to push a lever. However, simply transferring these laboratory taps into the home would be undesirable in terms of the atmosphere they create. New designs more appropriate for the home could either be based on the principle of the lever, or other principles, such as an electronic eye that follows hand movement.

Finally, industrial and academic involvement is needed in research and development on home care technology. Attempts were made in this study to identify such activities in the Netherlands. While no definitive data can be presented, the project gained a strong impression that neither industry nor academia, with a few striking exceptions, is greatly involved in home care technology. The sections that follow describe a number of potentially rewarding areas for development. However, the market for such developments is not clear in the present situation in the Netherlands. Without changes in the home care system itself, it seems unlikely that Dutch industry will find home care technology a good field for investment.

Section 3 – Some important Technologies not involving Equipment

The focus of this report - as far as technology is concerned - is on equipment, what is sometimes referred to as the 'hardware' of technology. Technology, however, also consists of 'software,' and in many instances that software is made up of human skills. Hardware without software is obviously absurd. Equipment is only useful if it supports human functions. On the other side, however, technology does not necessarily involve equipment. The purpose of this Section is to highlight a few **human** technologies that are important in home care.

Prevention

Influencing Life-styles. Aspects of individual behavior are related to important health problems, especially those patterns of behavior referred to as 'life style' (192;237). In the United States, it was estimated that as much as 50 percent of the mortality from the ten leading causes of death can be traced to life style (127). The situation is similar in the Netherlands. Known behavioral risk factors include cigarette smoking, excessive consumption of alcoholic beverages, use of illicit drugs, certain dietary habits, reckless driving, nonadherence to effective medication regimens, and maladaptive responses to social pressures (127;128). At the same time, a combination of genetic and environmental factors determines whether a particular individual will be affected, underlining the importance of an integrated prevention policy.

Methods of altering the burden of illness by changing behavior is a major issue in prevention (226;237). This involves information, communication, and motivation, often referred to as health education. More effective methods of health education may be developed and validated. Health education can be cost-effective, but each method will need to be analyzed carefully before social policy is made (202). The computer may have quite an impact in the area of personal behavior because of the availability of information from research findings, with dissemination through computer networks, and educational packages that can be developed for provider or individual use.

The Role of Stress. One problem is apparent, however. Unhealthy behavior is often the result of other factors, such as stress. People of lower socio-economic or cultural groups tend not to be reached by health promotion programs. Expecting people to change their behavior without addressing the factors that make their lives stressful and unsatisfying has been called 'blaming the victim.' Why do people behave in unhealthy ways? In particular, why do people of lower socio-economic status, who have poorer health than the general population, indulge in more unhealthy practices, such as smoking and excessive consumption of alcohol? It seems clear that powerful social forces influence these behaviors (22, p. 220). For example, people use smoking as a kind of coping behavior in stressful situations. Job stresses, divorce, family conflicts, loneliness, and other situations associated with anxiety and tension have all been reported to increase cigarette consumption. People who lack social and community contacts are more likely to be smokers (22, p. 221). Emphasizing life styles without also addressing social, economic, and environmental problems could be addressing symptoms instead of the real problems. It is probable that these non-health system factors are more important than life-style itself. In addition, social supports to help people through life crises and problems can be an important part of health promotion (see below) (237).

Nutrition

Nutrition is a major determinant of health. Consumption of foods that supply essential nutrients in adequate quantities and appropriate proportions is an absolute necessity for good health status.

The major societal problem in the area of nutrition in Western countries is how to develop and disseminate dietary recommendations based on current and future knowledge of human nutrition. Not only is this a difficult problem in itself, but it may be resisted by vested economic interests (such as those making and distributing dairy products). Nutrition policy needs to be active along the entire food chain, from production through marketing, to education of consumers of all age groups. Health education, briefly introduced above, is an important tool for helping people choose a healthy diet, an important part of home care, especially with regard to the elderly (113;202).

Screening and diagnosis are important techniques in determining the dietary requirements of the elderly. The nutrient needs and nutritional status of the elderly have only recently begun to attract the attention they merit. Dietary recommendations are largely based on studies of younger people (42). Throughout most of adult life, physiologic functions progressively decrease in efficiency. An important question is the extent to which life-style factors, notably nutrition and exercise in middle life as well as old age, can mitigate this erosion of tissue and organ function. The progressive reduction in energy intake occurring throughout adult life generally results in consumption of smaller amounts of nutrients (168;169).

Certain specific chronic diseases and disabilities are related to aging (168). These conditions include atherosclerosis, arthritis, and hypertension. Both human epidemiological studies and animal experiments on the process of aging suggest strongly that nutrition plays a role in the onset and development of these conditions.

It is unclear to what extent nutrition can reduce progressive age-related erosion of tissue structure and function as the adult grows older. Loss of bone mineral content resulting in osteoporosis is certainly influenced by dietary factors (see **brief**). Nutrition is also one of the major causative factors in age-related degenerative diseases such as atherosclerosis and cancer.

Because the nutritional needs of the older person have quite a considerable impact on health and well-being, assessment of nutritional status should be a routine part of every geriatric patient's initial examination, and all follow-up examinations as well (9).

Social and Psychological Supports

As already mentioned in the section on life-styles, perhaps one of the most striking areas of research is the growing body of evidence about the influence of social circumstances on health and functioning (80;127;237). For example, through-out the socioeconomic spectrum, men and women with few social contacts have higher mortality rates than those with many social connections (22, p. 217). Loss of a spouse or a child leads to a variety of problems, including even death (187). Crowding in urban areas is associated with stress, violence, and serious health problems.

Prevention and Treatment of Osteoporosis

Osteoporosis is a reduction in bone mass in the skeleton that increases susceptibility to fracture. It is the most common bone disorder in elderly women and a major public health problem (223). Almost all women over age 75 and about three-quarters of women over the age of 65 have osteoporosis of the spine (135). Fractures of the hip, vertebrae and distal radius (lower arm bone) are particularly common in individuals with osteoporosis. Hip fractures, especially, are important because they cause considerable disability and many premature deaths. Those who survive hip fractures often suffer permanent disability, and up to 25 percent remain in long term care institutions for at least one year after the fracture (57).

The relatively rapid rate of bone loss in middle-aged and older women is related to decreased production of estrogen (135). Low levels of dietary calcium are also associated with osteoporosis (168; 169), as have other factors, such as a lack of physical activity, a number of diseases, the intake of certain drugs, lack of Vitamin D, and excessive intake of alcohol, caffeine and nicotine. In elderly women protein intake can be reduced to prevent excessive calcium excretion. Fluoride is important in the remineralization of bone that has lost its calcium. The complexities in the development of osteoporosis are far from completely understood.

Both exercise and dietary precautions can affect the development of osteoporosis. There is some evidence that, besides physical activity, calcium intake during childhood and the teen years may be especially important (135). Calcium supplementation in the adult years appears to afford some protection. Calcium intake in postmenopausal women is particularly important (223). Estrogen loss with menopause leads to an increased need for calcium; it is recommended that the daily intake should rise from 800 mg to 1500 mg (46). The calcium content in diet can easily be increased by eating dairy products and leafy vegetables. Calcium salts can be used as supplements. Moderate physical activity, such as brisk walking every day, is also beneficial for the elderly. Intake of vitamin D and fluoride may also be protective, but are not entirely proven. For elderly women who remain indoors, a vitamin D suppletion may be considered.

Osteoporosis can, then, be prevented. But what about treatment? There is no validated screening procedure available, although CT scanning has been advocated by some. Once the problem is suspected and diagnosed, individual adjustments of diet, vitamin D intake, personal advise with respect to excercise and behavior and adaptation of the environment show excellent overall results. Considering present knowledge, intake of vitamin D and fluoride are only indicated under special circumstances.

The major problem is whether estrogen therapy should be given to postmenopausal women. Estrogen is effective in preventing bone loss, but may be associated with other health problems, including endometrial (uterine) cancer (46). There is now consensus that long-term cyclic estrogen suppletion in combination with progestagens has a considerable preventive effect without increasing the risk of endometrium cancer. However, studies of the long-term benefits and risks of estrogen in osteoporosis remain a priority. The implications of wide spread life-time intake of estrogen for all women at the menopause is as much a social as a medical question.

In summary, the diet of most people in Western countries probably contains insufficient calcium to prevent persistent net bone loss. As a minimum preventive measure for osteoporosis, all people should have an adequate calcium intake. Even more important is the lack of physical activity in industrialized countries. Exercise should be stimulated at all ages.

In the past, informal social networks supported people in stressful situations. However, social networks and social structures have been partially destroyed in industrialized countries in the course of the last and present century. As family, neighbours, and friends, and such institutions as the church, have become less important in dealing with people's problems in every-day living, a wide range of supports have become medicalized and professionalized.

Social and psychological supports may be developed to amelioriate and even prevent the effects of stress (79;134;159). Stress management techniques are being developed to help people handle the problem, particularly at work. Stress management can also assist in the rehabilitation of people with chronic diseases, such as those who have had myocardial infarction or heart operations (128). Higher levels of social support have been associated with moderation of the health consequences of unemployment, with lower mortality rates, and with health-related practices such as smoking, alcohol consumption, physical activity, obesity, and utilization of preventive health services (213).

These findings raise the possibility of active social interventions being developed and validated. Social supports have been found to reduce psychological stress following job loss or bereavement, to protect against depression after a major life event, and even to enhance recovery from severe burns (159). Creative health promotion and disease prevention programs in the future may integrate attention to life style, self-care, and social supports.

Self-care

Self-care refers to unorganized health activities and health-related decision-making by individuals, families, neighbours, friends, and colleagues (256). Although the definition of health care technology used in this report refers primarily to technology used in organized services, these services interact in various ways with self-care. Including this category in the report does not imply, however, that self-care should be supervised by professionals.

A part of self care concerns living a healthy life-style. This topic has been briefly discussed above.

Self-care also concerns therapy for the less complicated ills that may lead to visits to health services. Techniques should be developed to improve people's knowledge of when it is safe to care for themselves and when care by a professional might be more desirable. Many new technologies are becoming available to individuals for home use without professional supervision, and this trend will accelerate in the future (see sections that follow for such examples as home diagnostic kits, home supports, and computer systems, especially networking and monitoring).

In a time of increasing chronic disease (basically because of the aging of the population), the health services have an ever increasingly difficult time coping with the burden of providing care. At the same time, chronic disease offers many possibilities for self-care, both with and without the support of professionals. Self-care can take many forms. It can be a rejection of organized health care. It can be a creative personal response to the difficulties of finding ongoing support. Or it can be a partnership with professionals working in the organized health services (140).

For those suffering from chronic disease (diabetes, asthma, coronary artery disease, epilepsy, migraine), studies suggest that self-care is necessary even to realize limited medical goals (35;36). Understanding of the implications of the illness is essential if the person is to follow a healthy diet or take a medication consistently and in the appropriate dose. In this situation, the health care provider and the person with the chronic condition become partners in the care. In effect, the clinician becomes a consultant to turn to in case of need.

One study (175) examined the effectiveness of medical self-care education for elderly people. The investigators found improvements in health knowledge, in attempts to change life style, and in life quality. However, utilization of medical care and health status were unchanged.

Self-care has received rather little attention as a field or an activity. This situation seems to be changing (256). For reasons mentioned, self-care seems certain to grow in the future. It may offer a cost-effective model for ongoing patient care in the health services system, including in the home. It is certain that people **do** care for themselves; therefore, issues such as where to obtain information are critical. Self-care groups are growing in a number of countries. Perhaps governments could follow the positive social policy of encouraging and evaluating such activities, with the idea of supporting them more actively if they can be shown to have positive effects on the health status of populations.

Rehabilitation

People with disabling conditions or handicaps are particular candidates for home care services. Handicaps can result from congenital abnormalities, from diseases, or from injuries. An increasingly important cause of handicaps and functional problems is aging. As the average age of the population increases in Western countries, the prevalence of such problems is also increasing. Therefore, the emphasis of the technology should be on improving the functional autonomy of the person with the handicap. For the purposes of this part of the report, the cause of the handicap is less important.

Rehabilitation services have a great deal to offer in improving functioning, and future technology could offer additional possibilities. However, rehabilitation services need more emphasis and attention (136). This part of the report is addressed to the human services in rehabilitation; a later section will focus on devices and prostheses.

Rehabilitation refers to helping a disabled person gain the highest possible level of functional ability (183;255). It includes social and psychological elements, physical skills, and physical technologies. Rehabilitation could advance rapidly in the next few years, both through improved administration and coordination of services and through new technology. For an aging population, with a possible increase in physical problems, new models of rehabilitation will be needed (16). Holistic and multidisciplinary approaches may be critical in this respect.

Early discharge without adequate rehabilitation may reinforce disabilities, leading to further functional problems and increasing costs (8). Effective rehabilitation requires participation of the patient in decisions and encouragement to achieve independence (8;40).

Geriatric Rehabilitation is a set of mainly 'low' technology medical, nursing, social and remedial interventions provided for acute and subacutely ill elderly patients to help them attain their maximal functional independence (16). Elderly sick people must be evaluated early in the course of an illness and then must be furnished an appropriate set of services to assist them to reach their highest potential level of functioning. In general, this will require a multi-disciplinary set of services, including social work, nursing, physical therapy, and occupational therapy. This implies changes in the present pattern of services. Evaluation of the geriatric patient to assure appropriate services is a critical function (200). Special services of this type lead to improved outcomes for elderly people (8;40;154).

An aspect of disability in the elderly is the frequent occurrence of depression. Effective treatment of this condition is essential for rehabilitation and full functioning (145). Enriched environments may also be especially beneficial for elderly people (53).

Terminal Care. Terminally ill individuals have different medical needs from acutely ill patients, focusing on caring rather than curing (107;259). Rigorously applied hospital routines, such as frequent measuring of vital signs and restricted visiting hours, can make dying more uncomfortable and lonely for both patients and families (102). Acknowledgement of these shortcomings has prompted a search for more humane approaches and the emergence of programs designed exclusively for terminal care (3).

Though dying people can be cared for in a variety of settings, varying from a hospital-centered approach and day care programs to home care, the general concept or philosophy that is followed in this new approach is that of 'hospice'. Hospice can be defined as palliative and supportive care for terminally ill patients and their families, either directly or on a consulting basis with the patients physician and/or district nurse. The whole family is considered as the unit of care and care extends through the mourning process. Emphasis is placed on symptom control, to keep the patient as symptom-free as possible, allowing them to maintain control over their remaining lives. Hospice services therefore are meant to:

1. provide medical care for the control of symptoms such as pain and nausea;
2. concentrate on bedside nursing to provide comfort and close attention to easing physical distress and providing emotional support;
3. create an atmosphere of love and concern; and
4. focus on the family unit by teaching both the patient and family members to cope with the situation and by including them in the caring process (176).

Throughout a terminal illness, there is often an interplay between institutional and noninstitutional care. Often there are brief periods of time for which institutional care is needed to assess the changing medical needs and provide respite for the family. For most of the period, however, hospital care is not essential. Many, though not all, patients prefer the home over an institution for those periods.

A number of home hospice programs have been developed in the last two decades. Some originate in the hospital, others rely more on community-based home care. The services are interdisciplinary in nature. In addition to the care by a nurse and a physican, patients also require care of a social worker and to a lesser extent of a pharmacist, a psychologist, and a nutriologist (56). Volunteer services are an important component in all home hospice programs. Quality of life is the key element in home terminal care. It provides the patient with a familiar surrounding and the family with primary responsibility for the provision of care, facilitating the family-patient relationship.

Home hospice is often believed to be less expensive than hospitalization. This subject is discussed in Section 1.

Section 4 – Medical Technologies in the Home

As mentioned in other parts of this report, the historical trend regarding medical technology is to provide it as part of hospital services (13). In the past, it has seemed natural for the hospital to be the 'home' for high technology services. However, the expense of a day in the hospital has raised questions about this practice. At the same time, it is apparent that many diagnostic and therapeutic activities, especially in the area of chronic diseases, may possibly be carried out in the home in a safe and effective way, and in many cases patients prefer this alternative. Technological breakthroughs in such areas as miniaturization, new materials, and computers as process controllers now enable traditional clinical medical technologies to be provided outside the sheltered environment of the hospital (26).

This section will introduce a number of medical services that still are provided primarily in the hospital, but may in the future be an important part of home care. Unlike some of the technologies mentioned in other sections, the use of clinical medical technologies in the home heavily depends on availability of, and training by, professional medical personnel. Regular check-ups and other medical services, and availability in case of complications, make a coordinated and readily accessible medical system indispensable for these home services. Cooperation of physicians, nurses, the pharmacist, and the patient and his or her family is the primary condition for application of medical technology in the home. In the case of specialized treatments, a practice must have a high enough prevalence of the disorder to make training of clinicians feasible.

Diagnosis

Diagnosis is one of the most critical parts of medical practice. Diagnosis is the process of determining a patient's illness from his or her complaints and from other sources of information. Diagnosis has always been a part of home care. The physician or nurse visiting the home carries simple diagnostic tools, such as stethoscopes, thermometers, equipment for measuring blood pressure, and instruments for examining the eyes and ears. In addition, it is common to carry containers for collecting samples for examination later in a laboratory.

One major change that can be envisioned in the future is more diagnosis in the home using kits, either by a health care provider or by the patient him or herself. Recent advances in microbiology and biochemistry have led to technological developments which indicate an increased potential for home diagnostic tests that could be comparable in sensitivity and specificity to those performed in clinical laboratories (96;210). Advances in development and production of monoclonal antibodies have made such kits possible (see brief on monoclonal antibodies). The major advantage of using this type of test in diagnosis is that quite precise results can be obtained in a short time, without requiring extensive instrumentation. Their application may result in early rational management of patients, with elimination of unnecessary therapy and diagnostic tests. Overall, the quality of patient care and management could be improved and costs lowered as a result. Telecommunications could also make the information from such tests readily available to physicians and other providers in other sites.

Monoclonal Antibodies and Diagnostic Testing

Monoclonal antibodies are highly specific and completely homogenous antibodies to a particular substance. They are one of the first practical products of the biotechnology revolution. They promise in themselves to have dramatic impacts on clinical laboratory testing.

All animals respond to invasion by substances foreign to their body, called antigens, by producing antibodies, protein chains that bind to the specific antigen. While each antibody is formed specific to only one antigen, it has not been possible to produce pure antibodies before monoclonal antibody technology was developed. Nonetheless, with growing knowledge of immunology, antibodies have found ever-wider application in medicine. Still, such applications were hampered by the lack of access to pure antibodies.

Monoclonal antibodies are produced by a cell culture made up of cell cultures of hybrid cells that result from the fusion of myeloma cells (an antibody-producing tumor) and lymphocytes. The resulting hybrid cells, called hybridomas, grow permanently in cell culture and produce clones of highly specific and homogenous antibodies, called monoclonal antibodies. For the first time, pure antibodies can be obtained at reasonable cost. Monoclonal antibodies have wide potential applications. For example, in industry, they can be used in purification systems, in particular for proteins (179). They are also used in medical research, especially to characterize biologic substances, and experimentally in therapy, especially for cancer. The greatest immediate application in medicine, however, is in diagnosis.

Monoclonal antibodies make extremely sensitive tests possible. Even without monoclonal antibodies, many diagnostic tests have developed using antibodies. Assays, especially for hormones, already relied on antibodies, but many of these tests are becoming easier as well as more specific and sensitive because of the availability of monoclonal antibodies. In addition, many new tests can be developed. For example, certain cancers produce small amounts of certain proteins. Monoclonal antibodies make it possible to detect these proteins. Cancer cells and other tissues can be labelled using monoclonal antibodies for identification. Pathogens, such as bacteria, can be labelled and diagnosed in a few hours instead of the days previously required. Thus, new tests will be developed in the years to come.

By 1986, a growing number of tests based on monoclonal antibodies were coming into widespread use, e.g. kits for diagnosis of pregnancy and ovulation. Hybritech, a subdivision of Eli Lilly, has sixteen diagnostic kits based on monoclonal antibodies on the market. In addition, monoclonal antibodies are available from many companies for specific research purposes. But the major impact in the future will be on the diagnostic laboratory. By 1990, it is estimated that 50 percent of all tests in the diagnostic laboratory will be based on monoclonal antibodies (262). The immunoassay reagent market in Western Europe was estimated to be US$ 360 million in 1981 and will grow to US$ 600 million by 1990 (262).

The ease of carrying out many of the tests makes it possible to do them in the clinic, or even in the home. Already kits for the diagnosis of pregnancy based on monoclonal antibodies are being marketed directly to the public (see brief on home diagnostic kits).

In summary, monoclonal antibodies are a technology with many advantages. They are, however, also associated with social implications. Automation of the clinical laboratories in the 1960s and 1970s helped lead to a proliferation of diagnostic tests of uncertain utility. Monoclonal antibodies seem certain to be associated with the same problem.

Whether home diagnosis by lay people using kits is a beneficial practice or not is a major issue for the future (see **brief**). In many cases a physician will supervise their use, as in the case of diabetes. However, a number of kits will be marketed **directly** to the public. This move will promote autonomy, but it also has dangers. Lay people are not taught to perform tests nor to interpret their results. Furthermore, no test can be completely accurate. The implications of false positives and false negatives need to be carefully considered in terms of potential anxiety or reassurance, and the subsequent health care consequences

Clinical Monitoring

This section deals with monitoring of a person's biological functions through such means as diagnostic tests. It is also possible to monitor vital functions such as heart beat and respiration using electronic devices. This form of monitoring, which can be done from a remote site, is described in the Section dealing with telecommunications and computers.

Home Diagnostic Kits

Monoclonal antibodies have made simpler, cheaper, and more reliable diagnostic tests possible. There are many positive aspects to this development. This case concerns one application that raises significant problems.

Monoclonal antibodies make possible the development of diagnostic 'kits' for measuring or identifying certain biological substances. The first application in a widely available kit was for pregnancy testing. In this kit, female hormones associated with pregnancy are identified in a test easily done in the home. Such kits have now been marketed directly to the public, and increasingly, women are examining their own urine for signs of pregnancy rather than approaching health care services for this diagnostic aid. Also, a test for ovulation based on the same principle is available (luteinizing hormone levels rise in the urine 15 to 20 hours before ovulation). This test is used as an aid to more natural methods of contraception, such as avoidance or 'rhythm' methods and to increasing the probability of fertilization. These two tests seem to be positive developments, assuming that the tests are accurate, since they enhance personal autonomy. In addition, they allow privacy of decision-making in sensitive personal areas.

In the future, a number of tests will become available (210; 262). Some of these will be done to monitor an on-going condition, and will involve the supervision of a health care provider. Examples are monitoring the urine or blood sugar level in diabetes (already frequently done) and monitoring drug levels. Other tests will be done on the initiative of the person, without the involvement of a professional. Examples are tests for sexually transmitted diseases, beginning with gonorrhea and chlamydia, and for urinary tract infection (210). This category is associated with several important potential problems.

One serious problem concerns the sensitivity, specificity, and interpretation of tests. No test is fully accurate. Even the best test is associated with 5 to 10 percent of false positives and false negatives. Any rate would probably rise in a situation where the person doing the test has not been trained in technique and interpretation. A person with a disease who does a test and obtains a negative result may not then seek needed therapy. A person without a disease who obtains a positive result will then seek care from the organized system, possibly driving up costs.

An example of the problem is the pregnancy test. Manufacturers state that pregnancy testing kits are up to 99 percent accurate, and the U.S. Food and Drug Administration found an average accurate of above 97 percent (64). However, one study found that overall sensitivity was 56 percent, while specificity was 83 percent (64). If this result is consistent in other studies, it would mean that almost half of women who were pregnant would have a test result indicating lack of pregnancy, while 17 percent of those who were not pregnant would have a test indicating that they were pregnant.

Another problem concerns genetic testing. Companies in the United States are developing genetic tests in kits for direct sale to the public (122). While tests for such rare problems as Huntington's disease and cystic fibrosis will probably be available first, the large potential market is in more common conditions such as diabetes and heart disease. People could do a test, for example, and learn that they have a predisposition to coronary artery disease. The problem is that the implications of such information, even assuming that it is accurate, are not known. What is the probability of developing serious heart disease without changing diet and exercize habits, and following such change? Is the improvement worth the anxiety and concern produced in the person doing the test? Given the hundreds of genetic tests that will eventually be feasible, these questions are multiplied several times and present serious societal concerns. Nonetheless, in the long run, such tests offer significant potential for prevention of disease.

Diagnostic kits are entirely unregulated in the Netherlands, and in most European countries. There is no body to assure that tests offered to the public are in fact accurate when carried out by lay people. There is no body to determine when it is in the public interest to have direct access to tests and when not. This is a serious problem. Home diagnostic testing is certain to grow in the coming years (210).

As mentioned in the previous section, the treatment of chronic disease often requires self-care by the patient. It is not feasible to have a trained health care professional with every person having a chronic disease all of the time. Increasingly, people with certain chronic diseases are monitoring their own clinical status and adjust their therapy accordingly. Monitoring can also be done by different providers: relatively simple monitoring by family assistants, more complicated monitoring by nurses, and complicated disease monitoring by physicians.

Diabetes is the prototype condition for self monitoring with professional support and supervision (21;161;190). The morbidity of the disease can be reduced by 'tight' control of the blood sugar level (see **brief** on home care for diabetes). There is increasing evidence to suggest that meticulous control of blood glucose may delay or even prevent the microvascular complications of diabetes mellitus (214;218). A major barrier in the past was the limitation of urine glucose testing, the sole means available for a patient to self-monitor diabetic control. Technological advances, however, have made home monitoring increasingly attractive for diabetes.

Several manufacturers sell portable devices or chemically-treated test strips that the diabetic patient can use at home. Only a drop of blood is required; it can be produced by a fingerprick (78). The patient is able to check his or her blood sugar two to four times a day, and can adjust the amount of insulin needed accordingly. If necessary, consultation with the clinician by telephone can be used to check any decision. Home monitoring still requires frequent visits to the physician's office so that adjustments can be made and important trends can be identified by the physician (7;123). However, in the well-controlled diabetic, the number of clinic visits can be decreased.

A recent advance is insulin pump therapy in which insulin is infused by means of a small pump; this technique is impossible without blood glucose monitoring. Insulin pump therapy seems to have advantages for the control of some cases of diabetes (72;78). Improved treatment can prevent complications, and close monitoring by a health care professional is not required. The use of home testing therefore seems to be both beneficial and potentially cost-effective. In the future, biosensors may make this a more automatic process (151).

Home Care for Diabetes

It is known that people with diabetes develop fewer complications if the level of their blood sugar is closely monitored and controlled. Until recently, this required continually care by a professional. Technological advances, hwoever, have made home care increasingly attractive.

The technology has two components. One is a simple method for regular home monitoring of blood glucose levels. The other is a continuous insulin infusion by a small electromechanical pump worn on a belt or carried in a pocket (78).

Several manufacturers sell portable devices or chemically-treated test strips that the diabetic patient can use at home. Only a drop of blood is required; it can be produced by a fingerprick. The devices sell for US$250-400. Testing blood glucose at home for this purpose costs US$40-60 per month (72).

Use of the pump requires an initial period of stablization, probably in a hospital. Once an appropriate rate of insulin infusion is established, the pump is set to deliver insulin at that rate. The patient then checks the blood sugar at home two to four times a day, and can adjust the rate of insulin infusion. If necessarry, consultation with the clinician by telephone can be used to check any decision. A pump costs from US$900 to US$2,000. In addition, supplies are needed. It is estimated that using a pump costs US$2,000 a year, not including the cost of insulin, compared with US$200 for conventional syringes and supplies.

The use of home testing seems to be both beneficial and cost-effective. Improved treatment can prevent complications, and close monitoring by a health care professional is not required.

The insulin pump is not so clear, however. It has already found use in diabetic patients who could not achieve normal blood glucose levels by convential injection of insulin. Otherwise, the main advantage of the pump is that it is no longer necessary for the patient to inject insulin by needle multiple times a day. In addition, the patient on the pump has great flexibility in his or her diet and fewer symptoms from excessive or insufficient insulin. Otherwise, the benefits of the pump are not clear. Thus, the main known benefit is improvement in quality of life of the person with diabetes.

It is possible that biosensors may be developed that can automatically monitor blood sugar levels. In that case, a closed-loop system could be developed, in which a small computer automatically adjusted the level of insulin infusion. This would further improve quality of life.

Medical supervision continues to be important in home care for diabetic patients. Follow-up care is needed by clinical specialists, such as physicians and nurses. Assistance may be needed periodically in reprogramming the pump infusion rate. The patient must have ready access to clinical services accustomed to care for diabetes.

Thus, although home monitoring of blood sugar seems effective and cost-effective, it is not clear that use of the pump is money-saving. More experience and evaluation is needed to determine the answer to that question.

Another prevalent disease that can be monitored by the person with the disease is hypertension (high blood pressure). The technique required is simple; it takes about 20 minutes for a nurse to explain the principles and train the patient. Results can be used to modify treatment accordingly.

Treatment

Clinical therapeutic technologies as, for instance, parenteral nutrition, renal dialysis, and cancer chemotherapy, are becoming available for home care (see **Section 1** for data on costs of these technologies given in the home). Technological advances are making it safer to administer advanced therapies at home. Consumer-friendly, reliable, and durable technologies are being developed for home treatment. Infusion pumps are more trouble free, catheters for solution infusion have been improved, and more is known about patient responses to nutritional solutions. An increasing number of technologies is now considered to be potentially eligible for use in home care. The technologies discussed in this section have, more or less, been accepted for home applications. Others, varying from specialized burn treatments to certain orthopedic procedures, such as traction, are beginning to be explored for use in the home. This section gives but a selection of available clinical technologies. Not discussed are, for instance, urological products, bone growth stimulation devices, and transcutaneous electrical nerve stimulation (TENS).

Home Parenteral Nutrition (HPN). Home Parenteral Nutrition is the administration of an intravenous nutrient fluid to the patient at home (125;131). The technique was developed in the late 1960s for patients who had terminal intestinal failure and required permanent parenteral feeding (54;60). The three most common diagnoses found among patients on HPN are: inflammatory bowel disease; ischemic bowel infarction with resection; and malignancy-related gastrointestinal problems (131;251). HPN appears to be a (cost)effective alternative for cancer patients. They suffer much less morbidity from gastrointestinal complications of their malignancy.

HPN often is started by inserting a catheter into the vena cava (a vein in the abdomen). Hospitalization is needed for training the patient in the techniques of HPN. This must be done carefully and systematically in order to minimize subsequent complications. The instruction includes: information on the equipment and supplies; mixing of the solution with aseptic technique; care of the catheter; insertion of a heparin lock; administration of the fluid; and problem-solving techniques for therapeutic and equipment complications. After discharge from the hospital, the patients infuse their HPN solutions during a 10-12 hour period at night.

HPN allows patients independence and an acceptable quality of life (34;69;170;171). In HPN, the near-normal lifestyle with, for instance, high employment rates among patients is an additional (economical) incentive for widespread use of the technology. However, careful selection of patients is essential for success.

Drug Delivery Systems. Implantable reservoirs or pumps for drug therapy are already available, and are becoming an important part of this form of home care (49). The most widespread use at the moment is in diabetes treatment. Pumps are also currently used in cancer therapy (see below) and for the long-term administration of heparin in people with clotting or blood vessel problems (71). With improvements in the technology, pumps may spread into more widespread use, both for the indications listed and for other conditions. For example, continuous morphine can be infused in people with chronic pain (71).

Through the development of microelectronics, implantable micropumps will be used soon to deliver drugs continuously over extended periods (25), possibly leading to an expanded role in home care. A more distant possibility is the development of a 'biochip' or 'biosensor' which measures a biological variable or drug level in body fluids by combining microprocessors with biomedical instrumentation to monitor body parameters (37) (see also **brief** on pumps and biosensors in diabetes). The computer can be programmed to respond to a physiologic variable in addition to being governed by physical laws. Micropump technology is used to deliver a drug to alter or maintain the variable. The most obvious application here is the control of blood glucose in diabetics or administration of drugs with a small therapeutic window, e.g., anti-cancer agents or digoxin (25).

The Use of Pumps and Biosensors in Diabetes

Diabetes is a chronic disease characterized by insufficient insulin secretion and a resulting disorder of carbohydrate (sugar) metabolism, which can lead to serious complications such as kidney disease, vision problems, and nerve degeneration. It afflicts about 2 percent of the population, or about 300,000 people in the Netherlands. About 30,000 to 40,000 of these are dependent on insulin, that is, they must have an injection of insulin at least once a day (97).

In recent years, it has been realized that some of the complications of diabetes are prevented if the blood glucose (sugar) is kept close to normal (referred to as "tight control"). In the past, tight control was very difficult because of the difficulty of repeatedly doing tests of blood glucose and injecting insulin depending on the result. However, dry stick tests have made it easy for a person with diabetes to test the blood sugar at home. The most recent innovation is the insulin pump (continuous subcutaneous insulin infusion, or CSII), which the person wears on a belt or carries in a pocket. Insulin is infused continuously, and the amount can be adjusted by the patient (72;78).

Biosensors make it conceivable that this can be done automatically. Research on biosensors has led to the development of systems for reading the amount of glucose in the blood stream, but these have to be adjusted fairly frequently. If a stable biosensor can be developed, it could be combined with a small computer so as to make a system to speed up or slow down the infusion of insulin directly (a 'closed-loop system'). This technology seems possible within five years or so, but some experts are skeptical that it will ever become completely operational.

The problem is that the benefits of the pump are not well-understood. In addition, there are technical problems with existing pumps that keeps them from being completely reliable. At the same time, the quality of life of the patient is improved because there is no necessity for repeated needle punctures. But other health effects are uncertain. The pump is expensive, with an initial cost from Dfl. 2,500 to 5,000. A pump with an automatic feedback would probably be more expensive, although the cost will come down in time.

Industry is quite interested in the development of a closed-loop system, and has made considerable investment in this area.

The situation with diabetes is complex, since alternatives are developing, including pancreas transplant. These alternatives make chosing therapy more and more difficult.

Knowing whether or not to invest in this application of biosensors is a difficult problem for the future because of possible large aggregate costs and uncertain health benefits.

The measurement of drug levels in such a critical system is likely to be in the more distant future, beyond the year 2000, since analytical methods lag behind those of drug technology. In the future, as the ability to administer drugs through the skin increases and as it becomes easier to monitor blood levels of drugs, ever smaller devices will be designed to carry out these functions. Similarly, other body parameters, such as levels of enzymes and metabolites, will be monitored to allow adjustments in treatment. With such technological developments, controlled administration of drugs in the home seems certain to spread.

Cancer Chemotherapy. There is an increasing number of patients with remittent or progressive cancer. Most patients with metastatic disease need a palliative systemic treatment, e.g., intravenous cytotoxic cancer chemotherapy. The development of special vascular access procedures for regional adminstration to lessen systemic toxicity and the availibility of portable infusion pumps permit chemotherapy treatment schedules which better address tumor growth and the biology of cancer. Using new pump therapies that deliver measured doses of drugs, this treatment can be used in the home (211). The patient receives chemotherapy without excessive hospitalization, resulting in an improved quality of life.

Intravenous Antibiotics. The developments in drug delivery systems that enable home chemotherapy also can be applied for intravenous delivery of antibiotics. Diseases such as osteomyelitis, deep fungus infections, cystic fibrosis, and pneumonia, are often best managed with 4 weeks or more of intravenous antibiotic therapy (233). Home care programs can circumvent the inconvenient and expensive hospitalization for the therapy, provided that the patient is clinically stable and cooperative and that medical assistance is available at home. The presently used technique for intravenous antibiotic treatment is similar to that used for home parenteral nutrition and home administration of factor VIII and IX by hemophilia patients (141). The patient is catheterized and trained in the routines for intravenous antibiotic administration. During the program the catheter sites have to be changed every 2 to 3 days by a physician or (district) nurse. Several studies found home intravenous antibiotic therapy to be effective, safe, and cost-effective (see Section 1). In addition, the patients were much more comfortable at home, some of them even were able to return to work or school.

Management of Respiratory Failure. Patients with a variety of diseases and health problems require continuous support for breathing. Many of these patients have lung diseases such as chronic obstructive pulmonary disease (86). Others have poor or absent function of the muscles that make breathing impossible because of such problems as poliomyelitis, amyotrophic lateral sclerosis, and spinal cord injury (2;215;216). Still others need continous or intermittent oxygen therapy (188); in addition to lung conditions, serious heart diseases such as coronary artery disease also can fall into this category.

A variety of treatments can be provided in the home. Mechanical ventilators can support breathing, or can actually 'breathe' the patient who is unable to breathe on his or her own (68;101). Oxygen therapy can also be carried out in the home (87;110;156).

A new development that appears to have great promise for home oxygen therapy is devices to enrich the concentration of oxygen the patient breathes. Before these devices were invented, it was necessary to furnish oxygen in containers such as heavy metal bottles. Oxygen concentrators simplify this process and make it considerably cheaper.

Respiratory therapy can apparently be given at a lower cost in the home (see Section 1).

Renal Dialysis and Peritoneal Dialysis. For people with terminal renal failure, the only options are death, kidney transplant, or removal of poisons from their body by dialysis (83). Dialysis is the process of separating substances in solution by the differences in their rates of diffusion through a semipermeable membrane. Dialysis has several forms, but usually is done by hemodialysis, in which the blood from the patient's body flows through an 'artificial kidney', a dialysis device. Dialysis occurs through an artificial membrane between a blood compartment and a dialysate compartment. Both blood and dialysate flow through the artificial kidney by means of a pump system. Filtration is enhanced by exerting pressure on the blood passing through the membrane.

Dialysis can be done at home, and has been done at home since its very beginning (59;66;91). In some countries, more than 50 percent of those undergoing hemodialysis carry out the procedure themselves (with support) at home. As mentioned in Section 1, this procedure is cost-effective in societal terms (52).

A new technology now spreading into use is continuous ambulatory peritoneal dialysis (CAPD). In CAPD, the dialysis fluid is installed in the patient's abdomen through a catheter, and dialysis occurs across the membranes inside the abdomen. An agent such as glucose is added to the dialysate to enhance filtration. The procedure allows the patient to be fully ambulatory; dialysis occurs continuously, while the patient is at work or carrying out normal activities. By definition, CAPD is considered to be a form of home dialysis (146).

Section 5 – Technologies Adressed to Improving Functioning

In contrast to the previous section, focusing on traditionally clinical technologies moving into the home; this section addresses new and improved technology that enhance the capacity of people with functional limitations to take care of themselves (153).

The prevalence of functional problems in most industrialized countries is significant. Approximately 15 percent of the Dutch population has limitations of activity from chronic conditions such as heart disease, arthritis and rheumatism, perceptual disorders, hypertension, and impairments of the back, spine, lower extremities or hips. As these conditions are correlated with aging, their prevalence can be expected to rise in future. Especially in elderly people, multiple disabilities often exist at the same time, this has important consequences for future technological design. Existing technologies often are designed in response to particular disabilities. However, as Orleans and Orleans (186) note: ". . . this focus on the unique problems of specialized groups impedes our examination of the common performance limitations that occur in all populations and among all people at particular times and under special circumstances throughout their lives." The area of technologies for functioning is hampered by lack of definition of needs, lack of criteria for design, and lack of clear indication of which tools would improve the functional environment.

Both the mental and physical chronic health problems can be categorized as to their resulting performance limitations. Steinfield and Hiatt (229) have developed a list of such common performance limitations (see Section 1). Experience in the Netherlands is consistent with this list. The Technical University of Eindhoven has found that a particularly critical problem is body support during standing, kneeling, or sitting. Changing position, for example for those in a wheelchair, can be a signficant problem. Movement, particularly to go to the toilet, is another common problem.

Many technological innovations can increase the social and physical mobility and functioning of the elderly and handicapped. Rehabilitation services and new forms of rehabilitation will aid in this shift toward encouraging autonomy. Traditionally, rehabilitation has not been accorded great importance in relation to other activities of the health care system (153). The focus of the health care system has been on diagnosis and therapy. However, as long term handicapping conditions are becoming more prevalent, and are leading to higher expenditures for society, interest in functional technologies that address above mentioned limitations will increase.

In providing future technological support, two basic strategies can be followed:

1. technologies can be directed towards the functional limitation itself, e.g. as in prosthetics; or
2. technologies can be directed towards adjusting the environment, such as in height adjustable kitchen counters. This Section will be primarily addressed to technologies in category 1. However, the importance of engineering and environmental controls must not be forgotten. Environmental controls are particularly directed toward safety, as with smoke alarms and attempting to prevent falls.

Technology and Daily Living

Assistive devices can be used to compensate for functional impairment. Many technologies that enhance the activities of daily living are low-technology, such as long handled soapers for bathing, reachers and grippers to dress, clothes that open in front, adjusted kitchen utensils, as well as services such as meals-on-wheels. A large number of these technologies are directed towards improving safety in the home; e.g. non-skid floor materials; illumination systems reducing the amount of glare; appropriate designed stairways, and so forth. New and improved assistive devices and adjustments of the home environment will be spurred by developments in materials science. The area of materials science is evolving rapidly, with the coming of age of new polymers, metals, ceramics, types of glass, and composites containing new reinforcing fibers.

Many assistive devices have been developed but are as yet not widely used because they are not widely known, too expensive, or difficult to purchase; others are still in the early developmental phase. An additional problem is that often the relative small market permits only limited research and development efforts by industry (232).

Developments in high-technology concern mainly communication-technology. Hardness of hearing is a severe handicap, especially for social activities. There is a great need of devices that solve the problems concerning background noise versus orientation at conversation. Miniaturization and developments in processing of signals will bring solutions in this field. Telecommunications, spur the introduction of a whole range of new assistive devices. These technologies wil be discussed in the next section. Alas, assistive devices are generally not very ergonomic; that is, they have not been designed so that they are easy and comfortable to use. The Technical University of Delft studies the possibilities of improved industrial design by incorporating average sizes of the population.

A special category of assistive devices concern those which can be developed for mentally impaired individuals. These may include new memory training techniques: labels on objects, illustrated with simple drawings to clarify use, or clock radio systems that verbalize reminders.

Assistive devices can also be based on high technology. For instance, micro-electronics can not only be applied in communications but also to take over daily chores such as opening doors, picking up the telephone, and switching on the television or radio. A number of Dutch firms and institutes have developed such control devices. The Technical University of Eindhoven, for instance, has developed an electronic device that can be programmed for such tasks as turning lights, television sets, and heating systems on and off. The Swedish firm Permobil has marketed a similar communication system that can be mounted on a wheel-chair.

One interesting advance is the development in **robotics**. A robot is an automatic apparatus or device that performs functions ordinarily ascribed to human beings, or operates with what appears to be almost human intelligence. Design of robots has progressed rapidly in the past few years. They have been used for a number of areas in industries such as metal-working and automobile manufacturing. Knowledge on the mechanics of movement and the engineering of parts, the availability of micro-computers, and the development of sophisticated software is also leading to sophisticted robots for a variety of other purposes. A Dutch initiative in this respect is the development of manipulators that can be attached to a wheelchair by the Institute on Rehabilitation Issues (IRV). One type of robot is a 'nurse,' which can assist bedridden patients (77). While these robots will probably be used first in hospitals and institutions, they could also be used in the home, although applications seem years away. Both the sensory capabilities of robots and their ability to deal with unexpected events are still rather limited. Since the household environment varies greatly from one setting to another, robot command languages and sensing abilities will need to be improved (51). In the long run, it may be possible to design robots for a broad spectrum of daily chores such as opening doors, picking up the telephone, and switching on the television or radio. Work in voice recognition could lead to robots and other types of devices that respond directly to voice commands.

Prosthetics

The rapid pace of advance in the fields of micro-electronics, computers, understanding of nerve and muscle control, bioengineering knowledge of the dynamics of human movement, materials sciences, and the neurosciences, will result in far more sophisticated prostheses (103; 178). One of the main objectives will be to develop prosthetic devices that effectively replace defective parts of the human nervous system. Neurological prostheses are defined as wholly or partly implanted devices which stimulate nerve fibres or nerve cells electrically and thereby restore functions of the nervous system that have been lost as a result of disease or injury. This approach has already been used in spinal cord stimulation as a treatment for pain and spasms, and may also be used in neurologically derived problems of sexual functioning in men.

In the area of communicative disorders a number of new and future prosthetics can be anticipated. New and improved implantable or portable sensory aids for hearing, touch, speech, vision, and even smell may be developed (70;178), resulting from increasing the ability to electrically stimulate individual sensory nerves, selective parts of the spinal cord, and areas on the surface or within the brain. Indispensable to these abilities will be concomitant progress in microprocessor development as well as advances in the theories of signal processing to emulate sight and hearing (51).

Speech control devices will use computer-generated speech which will be directly controlled by the central nervous system (178). In the area of vision, lens implants can be anticipated, which are inflatable or variable in power. This means that a smaller incision will be needed during cataract surgery. Furthermore, with children the power of the lens could be adjusted as the eyes change size.

New materials for oxygen permeable contact lenses will reduce current complications. Another development concerns visual devices which use direct cortical stimulation. Visual signal eye prosthetics and the possibility of the artificial eye will, however, need a real breakthrough to become viable (180).

The area of human movement is another area with a high future technological potential. Movement aids, wheel chairs, lifts for patients, and exercize systems can all be expected to improve. Advances further in the future include movement control systems, which use signals from peripheral nerves and/or spinal roots to control artificial limbs in amputees (240). Furthermore, the continuous advances with new, lighter and more durable materials will improve the problem of interfacing prosthetic devices with the patient's skin. A whole family of aids and prosthetics incorporating biofeedback may be possible. However, many problems must be solved first, including the difficulties of producing specific stimuli through nerves to implanted prostheses.

Functional electrical stimulation is a promising technology that is beginning to show results (103; 242). It is a particular focus of attention at the Technical University of Twente. The basic technique relates to electrical activation of innervated skeletal muscle as a means of affecting movement. The primary goal is to provide useful movements of the upper and lower extremities in persons with paralysis due to trauma or disease. Functional electrical stimulation is already an accepted clinical procedure for the treatment of idiopathic scoliosis, upper and lower extremity function in hemiplegia due to stroke, and in certain respiratory disorders. Its use as a long term assistive aid in paralysis has yet to reach the stage of clinical application. This is due to a number of factors including:

1. Implant devices rather then surface stimulators will be required for long term use. Such devices will require many channels in order to stimulate a large number of muscle groups and will have to incorporate advanced microprocessor technology to permit setting and control of many parameters and signals. Both the biomaterial and electronic design problems are great, but fast moving advances in technology suggest that these problems will be solved in 4 to 6 years.
2. Electrodes that exist today have many problems. It is still not clear whether the muscle (motor point nerves) or the peripheral nerve should be stimulated and with what form of electrode this should be done. Present research promises to resolve these questions within a few years.

3. Control systems that duplicate the complex function of the neuromuscular system have yet to be perfected. Their design requires an understanding of how the normal body is able to position the extremities, maintain balance, and control timing and force. Again, present research has produced many useful results and should provide the basis for clinically useful devices in 4 to 6 years, but these systems will be rudimentary and it will be many years before the more sophisticated human activities like running or dancing could even be contemplated.

Another area of prosthetics concerns itself with incontinence (84). Urinary incontinence is a prevalent problem, which is potentially (socially) disabling and costly to the health care system. Several types of incontinence exist. Present-day treatments include artificial sphincters, electrical stimulators, drugs, training procedures, and surgery. The artificial sphincter is a prosthetic device for those patients with severe incontinence caused by dysfunction of the bladder outlet and/or urethral closure mechanisms (182). Improvements in mechanical properties could increase the success rate and diminish complications of these devices. Another new development includes conditional pudendal nerve stimulators for biofeedback for treating urinary incontinence due to detrusor muscle instability. At present, sacral anterior root stimulators for controlling the urinary bladder are not very widely applied. In the coming years, they could become more successful and applied to a larger group of patients.

Section 6 – Telecommunications and Computers in Home Care

This Section concerns information technology, which involves the application of computers and telecommunication systems for the creation, storage, manipulation, and dissemination of information (20; 184). While advances within information technology could well have been presented in other sections - e.g. clinical monitoring as part of medical technology in the home, or remote shopping under technologies addressed to improving functioning - this area of technological change was singled out because of its anticipated pervasive influence in a wide variety of home care activities (158).

The main possible effect of telecommunications and computers in home health care is that all parts of the system, including the individual in his or her own home, can be linked into one network. A precondition for successful use of telecommunication in health care is the existance of such a system.

In a simplified form, the three major information flows are depicted in figure 2. An organization of this section is based on these three flows: a) within the individuals home and from the home to his or her personal environment; b) the interactive communication process between the home and health services; and c) information exchange within the health care system. The paragraphs dealing with communication between the home and health services focus especially on clinical information, while those dealing with information exchange within the health care system also include the administrative and organizational use of information technologies. The latter technologies might be considered to be 'process' technologies or technological applications that serve to support or organize the delivery of professional home health care.

Information Technology within the Individual's Home

In the coming decades computers and telecommunication technology are expected to move progressively into the individual's home (115). One application of information technology is to monitor different household functions, such as heating or electrical uses. For example: a 'sensaphone' is a system using microprocessors linked to one or more telephones, to gather and monitor information provided by sensors

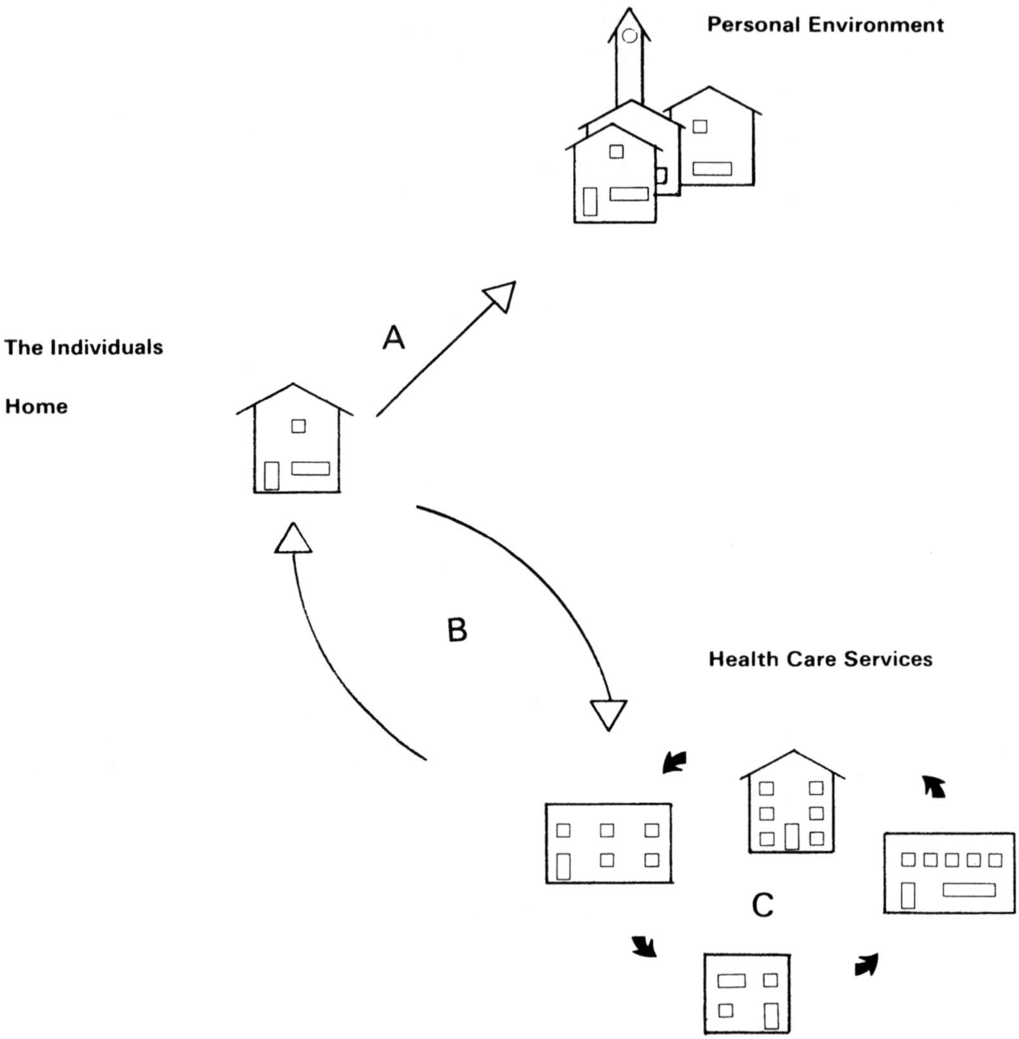

Figure 2 Information flows in home health care

located throughout the house. Based on this information, remote control (by the individual in the house or by care individuals outside the house) of all household activities can be envisioned. For example, Nixdorff two years ago installed a full-fledged computerized 'home' as a laboratory setting to experiment with age-specific household functions. Another application within the house concerns the use of wake-up services, pre-programmed to remind the individual of medication times.

An important aspect of information technology is the exchange of information with the personal environment. Remote shopping and banking, for instance, are expected to increase in the future and can enhance the capability of people to care for themselves. With an increasingly elderly and sometimes frail population, the availability of alarm systems is of importance, not only in terms of physical health but also in terms of an increased sense of security. Information technology leads to the development of different kinds of new alarm systems, which in case of emergencies are used to alert friends or relatives outside of the house or at a central monitory centre. These alarm systems can be used in conjunction with special detectors locating the person for instance within the city (see also brief).

Of course, the telephone is the major communication device. Computers can be readily hooked into the telephone system for health care purposes. In the long-run, video telephones may become widespread, enhancing communication possibilities.

Personal Alarm Systems

One major problem preventing older and handicapped people from staying alone in the home is that they might not be able to call for help if needed. This problem can be addressed by a personal emergency response system (PERS). A PERS is a signalling device that employs a portable transmitter (remote activator) to activate a receiving base (the home communicator unit), which in turn summons help through the telephone system (76). In both cases, the user carries a small, wireless transmitter around the neck, on the belt, on the wrist, or in a pocket. When an emergency occurs, the person presses a button. The button sets off a response that either alerts a responder directly or alerts an emergency monitoring center that communicates with the responder (an ambulance system, for example).

A wide range of emergencies can be addressed by a PERS system:
1. Such medical conditions as heart attack or diabetic shock;
2. Inability to get up after a fall, such as out of bed;
3. The presence of an intruder, the smell of smoke or gas, the loss of electricity; and
4. Momentary disorientation, panic attacks, and acute spells of loneliness (76)

In the United States, systems have developed to provide the back-up for home monitoring. The major system in the U.S. provides a starter package for 20 subscribers for US$15,000. Typical monthly subscriber fees are US$15 to US$30 (76).

In the Netherlands, such systems are available in several cities, including Breda and Amsterdam.

Information Exchange between the Home and Health Services

A general principle must be kept in mind in organizing health services: the main purpose of services is care. Computers and telecommunications cannot replace people. They can only be used to enhance and support personal care.

In a general sense, networks of computers between institutions, health care workers, and private individuals will permit a continuous flow of information, with feedback (225). Home care of patients with acute myocardial infarction may, in some cases, be advantageous. For example, people will progressively be able to use preventive, diagnostic, monitoring, and therapeutic possibilities at home which are now only available in hospitals and institutions and by consultation with professionals. They may be able to measure and monitor their own blood pressure, blood sugar, and so forth. They will have access to their own medical data and to computerized information and advisory services. This will make the population less dependent on institutional care and cure, and can create more autonomous decision making.

In general, with the increased number of personal computers, new possibilities excist to provide health education and disease prevention. Educational packages can be developed for specific health related problems or for certain disorders. While these activities concern general information exchange, person to person exchange with the health care provider will also increase.

The computer, in association with other advances, such as those in telecommunications, is changing the concept of monitoring vastly. Within many health care institutions computer-assisted monitoring is expanding greatly. For example, monitoring of blood gases for those with respiratory failure or after surgery could become routine through miniaturization.

The trends towards simplification and portability of equipment in health care technology will enable monitoring functions to move to clinics and also to people's homes. The first change will be to move certain functions to clinics. Subsequently, home monitoring will become increasingly implemented (74; 261). In many cases, however, monitoring will be done to communicate vital signs of a patient to a clinic or physician's office (39; 55). Furthermore, computerized monitoring can be important in measuring progress in chronic problems. In return, the patient can receive information from the health care provider in the form of health instructions or pharmaceutical instructions. In any monitoring, however, a great deal of attention must be given to minimizing false positive and false negatives.

These interactive systems of medical monitoring can be designed in a variety of ways:

a. a computer periodically calls patients and prints out routine questions;
b. the concept of the 'hospital on the wrist,' including a computer, a microminiature analyzer, and a drug reservoir with electronic probes capable of monitoring changes in vital body signs and comparing these with expected values for the individual wearing it. However, such systems are still mainly in their research phase and are not yet available for routine use.

The development of expert systems for clinical use is an important computer application (247). Expert systems are programs developed by multidisciplinary groups of experts for problem solving, with the help of a system engineer to translate their expertise into machine language (150). These expert systems can be used both for computer assisted diagnosis and computer assisted therapy.

There are many obstacles to developing computer diagnosis, including imprecise medical terminology, use of nonindependent clinical parameters, incorrect or inaccurate information supplied to the computer, and static representation of the patient's medical record. Current applications have remained largely as experimental systems in research (257). In the coming years this situation will change as the difficulties involved will be addressed. In therapy, protocols for an acceptable quality of treatment can be developed and made available by computer (120). Such a system can translate clinical research and treatment protocols into a format which can be used on a computer and which permits a community physician or researcher to accurately follow a formal protocol or state-of-the-art regimen, to gather data, to order required tests, to order dosages at levels prescribed by the protocol or suggested by a panel of experts, and to schedule patient visits. A protocol requires making medical knowledge explicit and testing it critically against reality, with the final goal to make knowledge and experience more accessible in a number of areas in medicine. A protocol consists of treatment advice applicable in particular situations. When a situation is present, a patient's complaint for instance, a special protocol applied to the situation can be selected.

With the developments in artificial intelligence, the simulation or imitation of human intelligence by machines, it may be possible that computer assisted diagnosis and computer assisted therapy will spread. Work on artificial intelligence may make such systems more effective in the future (1; 27). It could be used by lay people at home. However, except in special circumstances, such developments seem years in the future. In particular, the problem of false positive and false negatives is likely to prevent widespread use of such systems at the community level.

Information Exchange within the Health Care System

In the coming years huge mass memories (e.g. on laser discs) for the storage of medical records and data can be expected to become widespread. Apart from storage in central mass memories, medical data will be recorded and stored in data bases both in hospitals and the offices of primary health care providers. This implies that different communication networks will develop between the various health care providers, including national or regional systems, not only for epidemiological studies, planning, managements, and evaluation, but also for consultation (167). Electronic archives will be installed for pictures, biological signals, and many other data. Extensive networks to provide expert specialist advice to home health care providers such as nurses and general practitioners seem very likely. Those who provide services in the home, such as nurses or general practitioners, could have ready access to such advice. Such advice could also be made directly available to the lay public.

Information on Available Assistive Aids and Devices

At present, information on available devices for home health care is sadly lacking. Ideally, a health care provider would carry out a needs assessment and then identify the most appropriate device. Alternatively, a person with a functional disorder may attempt him or herself to find a useful device. However, for the most part there is not even a list of available devices. When devices are listed, there is little evaluative information given, such as who can be expected to benefit or how reliable or difficult to use the device is.

A useful basis for information systems that are developing is the International Classification of Impairments, Disabilities, and Handicaps (ICIDH). It allows devices to be matched to a specific disability. However, many functional problems, such as problems reaching, are not so specific. Devices will be harder to classify in such cases.

In the Netherlands, there are a number of systems of information. These systems generally have little evaluative information on specific devices.

1. A rational project (NIG) collects information on where to obtain lists and evaluations of available aids and devices. This information is accessible to consumers. NIG does not itself have the information.
2. A national information system for handicapped people (IDC) has been developed on an experimental basis, with aids as one field of interest. IDC and NIG are considering merging their operations.
3. The Regionaal Informatiecentrum (RIC) Hoensbroek has information on available devices and runs expositions to demonstrate aids. It also published a newsletter on recent developments. RIC is part of a larger European project, the Handinet system, sponsored by the EC. It has rather complete lists of devices available for handicaps, but it lacks evaluative information.
4. The publishing firm Samson publishes a list of available aids (the PRIS), in cooperation with the Council of the Handicapped (Gehandicaptenraad). Samson also publishes leaflets with more detailed information on specific aids in cooperation with GMD and RIC.

5. Available information is primarily related to aids for specific handicaps, and often is only available through associations or regional centers that deal with that particular handicap. For example, information on communication disorders and devices for hearing and visual handicaps is relatively available.
6. The Stichting Warenonderzoek Gehandicapten has literature about specific aids, focusing on evaluation. In some cases, SWG funds evaluations itself. It also publishes materials that present such evaluative information.

As previously noted, lists of devices addressed to functioning, and especially devices that might be useful for elderly people, are less available. GMD has its own information system that is useful for this purpose.

Modern computers and telecommunications could make such lists quite accessible, even to people in their own homes.

Section 7 – Conclusions

Home care has much to offer. Many people with health problems or problems of every-day functioning can live relatively normal lives at home with a degree of support. An important effect of home care, then, is to improve the quality of life of people with chronic illness or disability. Technologies have considerable potential in improving such supports. Technology addressed to true health or functional needs has the additional advantage of offering industry possibilities for new activities.

At the same time, however, home care has not developed rapidly, and home care technology development and use has been correspondingly hampered. The existing 'system' of home health care in the Netherlands is fragmented, underfunded, and uncoordinated. Without significant and ongoing changes in this 'system', people's needs will not be fully met and technology will not reach its full potential.

Conclusion 1. Home health care in the Netherlands urgently needs organization

As described in this report, a number of different professions deliver care in the home. They are usually associated with different organizations and they obtain their payment in different ways. This multi-disciplinary approach requires very good coordination to maximize efficiency and benefit to recipients of the services. Mechanisms to assure this coordination are presently lacking.

In the long-run, new organizational approaches to home care are needed. It is difficult, given the complexity of the field and present changes underway, to draw a blue-print for such an organization. However, it is possible to lay out general steps toward accomplishing the aims described in this report:

1. More needs to be known about the implications of the use of machines in the home. What is the attitude of the public? What types of education are needed for best functioning of technology in the home? Are there other implications of technology in the home, such as making care less flexible or human?

2. More information must be gathered on the **needs** of people for home care. For example, little is presently known concerning the rates and severity of various functional problems in the elderly now and in the future.
3. Despite these limitations of knowledge, enough is known to begin to develop a better system. In time, with expanded information on needs, it is necessary to consider specific alternative organizational structures for home care. This requires the development of detailed **policy options** or **scenarios** putting together needs, personnel, and alternative organizational developments, including sources of payment. The costs of each alternative could then be detailed.
4. Pilot programs could be developed and evaluated in the field. This would give valuable experience and guidance for future action.
5. Ultimately, one comprehensive system could evolve from such efforts.

A number of different groups could perform the first steps. One reasonable possibility would be that the Steering Committee on Future Health Scenarios (STG) takes the initiative to develop scenarios concerning the future of home health care in the Netherlands. The scenario on cancer in the future supported by the STG is an example (238). The STG has already began a preliminary scenario on first line care. Perhaps home care could be part of that scenario.

Clearly, the Ministry of Welfare, Health, and Cultural Affairs (WVC) must take a leadership role in implementing changes in home health care. The Ministry could expand its support for pilot projects now. It could also commission and support research, such as epidemiological research on needs for home health care.

Ultimately, of course, the decisions that must be made are political.

Conclusion 2. One urgent problem in the organization of home health care is the lack of one professional with the main responsibility for assessing patient needs for home care and assuring that needed services are provided by the appropriate organization or care provider.

To make an analogy with drugs, society has assigned physicians the role of diagnosing disease and making prescription of appropriate pharmaceutical treatments. Such drugs generally cannot be obtained without such prescription, and insurance companies and sick funds will not pay for drugs without such a prescription. The requirement for a prescription both protects the patient from inappropriate treatments and protects the third party payor from inappropriate costs.

The same situation could be said to relate to home care technology. Only in the area of devices for the handicapped is this situation partially addressed (through the GMD). At the moment, little sophisticated technology is provided in the home. Part of the problem is that generally no professional is empowered to prescribe such technology. Another part of the problem is that third parties generally do not pay for the technology or pay only part. In addition, present incentives do not encourage home care, for example, by general practitioners.

In this report, no conclusion is reached as to which professional should serve this role. Some feel that the general practitioner already plays a key role in this area and should have this role strengthened. Others feel that nurses are closer to the home situation and could make a more realistic assessment. Still others feel that home care problems are often social or psychological in nature and that social workers should be the key professional. It does seem clear that whenever the patient has a medical problem, that problem should be assessed by a physician. In the case of handicapped people under the age of 65, the GMD already does a needs assessment and provides necessary devices and equipment. Otherwise, new organizations and differently trained personnel would be needed to for this expanded role.

Conclusion 3. Professionals involved in home care need specific training in the roles and tasks involved in such care. Specifically, they need to be oriented to available and future technology and to its evaluation.

As noted above, no one professional has the task of assessing patient needs and provided needed services and technology in the home. At present, no professional has appropriate training for this role. If such a role were envisaged, training in accord with this role would be needed.

In any case, home care seems certain to expand in the future, requiring that all of those involved in such care will need more specific training. Improved training and increased payment would increase the social status of this important activity as well.

Conclusion 4. If changes in the organization of home health care can make it more integrated and comprehensive, a vigorous market for home care technology will develop and industry will probably greatly expand its efforts in this area. With such changes, industry would find attractive incentives to enter the home care field.

When a market for technology is readily identifiable, as in the case of hospital care, industry has the capability to become rapidly involved. In the Netherlands, such a development would be beneficial both from the standpoint of providing improved home care and from an economic perspective (developing new jobs, increasing exports).

There is a role for government to stimulate the development of devices and equipment for home care, but such efforts will be most effective following changes in the organization of home care.

In developing home care technology, the most constructive approach will generally be to develop products that will also serve a general market. If products are attractive, simple to operate, and esthetic, they can often find such a wider market. For example, kitchen equipment can be designed for easier use by anyone. Remote control of electrical devices, lights, and heating could be attractive to many people. Even young people may have problems in reaching high shelves or lifting heavy objects.

The Netherlands market is generally a small one. This means that industry must be attentive to the possibilities in the international market place for home care technology.

Conclusion 5. Special attention needs to be paid to the relations between people and devices used in the home (the 'man-machine interface')

Obviously, equipment used in the home is not subject to continual professional monitoring. There could be quite long periods of time when the equipment is used by the recipient without supervision from a professional. This means that equipment used in the home, especially when it is a medical device addressed to a serious health problem, needs to be specially designed for easy use. It also needs to be particularly reliable.

Little is known about the effects of equipment use in the home, especially medical equipment such as dialysis machines and respirators. Well-designed studies of the implications of such use, the selection of patients, and the human supports necessary for effective use are needed. It may be, for example, that the life-long use of medical equipment will have severe emotional costs that will require special supports.

Most device failures in the home, whether of medical devices or devices addressed to functioning, are due to human error. This points up the need for careful selection of patients and for their orientation and training in their own care, since the support systems found in an institution cannot be provided in the home. Little attention has been paid to designing devices to avoid errors in use, and it seldom takes into account the fact that people receiving home care may have such problems as problems seeing or lack of strength. Presently available equipment is often difficult to use, even for those without functional problems.

Mechanisms are presently lacking for maintenance and spare parts of equipment used in the home, and are needed if such technology is to spread.

At present, medical devices are generally not regulated in the Netherlands. Attention needs to be given to mechanisms to assure needed reliability in this case.

Conclusion 6. There is an urgent need for information systems on available devices, including their cost, where they can be obtained, and the situations in which they are most useful.

Presently, available information systems are primarily oriented to specific handicaps, such as communication disorders. Such information systems are small and may be difficult to locate. Information systems on devices addressed to general functional problems are usually non-existent at present. In addition, all information systems have limited evaluative information.

Information systems are beginning to be developed and coordinated in this area both in the Netherlands and at the European level. Such developments need to be stimulated and supported.

Home care is a rather neglected field that seems likely to grow rapidly in the future. The greatest goal of home care is to promote autonomy of the patient. The most important task is to provide human services that can support such autonomy. At the same time, sophisticated technology can contribute to this goal, especially by promoting human care and allowing increased autonomy. Systems that work to provide appropriate technology to people in their home seem good for all parties - patients, those who pay for health care, industry, and government.

Appendixes

APPENDIX A   METHOD OF THE PROJECT

The need for examining future health care technology was recognized by the Dutch Steering Committee on Future Health Scenarios (STG) in 1984. (The STG is an independent advisory group to the Dutch government set up in 1983 to carry out scenario studies as an aid to long-term health planning). The STG initiated the Project on Future Health Care Technology. The World Health Organization, European Office (EURO), agreed to support the project financially and logistically.

The project had two specific objectives:
1. To identify future technological developments in health care, with brief descriptions of potential technologies; and
2. To carry out prospective assessments of four high priority technologies or areas of technological development.

The project began in April 1985. A Commission on Future Health Care Technology made up of 10 members and 5 official observers was appointed to guide the project. Surveys of experts were carried out in the United States and Europe. The information from the surveys, supplemented by material from the scientific literature and from interviews, was the basis for the overall descriptions of health care technology. The assistance of these many individuals and groups is specifically acknowledged in appendixes to Volumes I and II of this report.

The project plan called for four technologies to be prospectively assessed. In September 1985, the Commission met and endorsed four cases:
1. implications of neurosciences;
2. biotechnology probably examining both monoclonal antibodies and vaccines;
3. laser applications, especially in surgery and in the treatment of vascular disease, especially coronary artery disease; and
4. genetic screening and diagnosis.

Later, with funding from the Ministry of Economic Affairs, medical imaging and home care technology were also developed as case studies.

A detailed description of methods for the entire project is presented in an appendix to Volume I of the report. An updated version may be found in Volume II. And each case study contains a methods description specific to that case.

Material was collected on home care technology early in the project since the subject was covered as part of the overall description of health care technology (Volume II). During the fall of 1986, information gathering efforts were intensified and interviews were held with a number of experts in home care and technology. The efforts continued during early 1987.

NIVEL had applied to the Ministry of WVC for support of a project concerning technology for primary care. Ministry staff suggested that NIVEL and the project work together, and this was agreed. (NIVEL received the support for its own project.) Dr. Peter Groenewegen of the NIVEl staff agreed to draft a paper describing the home care system of the Netherlands. The paper was presented to the project, discussed, and revised. It was then sent to about 20 people either involved in home care or who had done research on home care. Based on their comments and criticisms, the paper was revised again, and became the basis for Section 2 of this report. Information on the availability of devices from the loan desks of the Cross-work organization was acquired for the project by a staff member of TNO and was added to this Section. Analysis of all of the material in this Section was done by project staff.

During April and May of 1987, drafting on the remainder of the report was carried out. The draft was then distributed to two working groups. A special working group met on 10 June to discuss the sections of the draft dealing specifically with home care and with the home care system of the Netherlands. Another working group met on 16 June to discuss the sections of the draft dealing specifically with technologies in home care. Both groups also reviewed and discussed draft policy options.

Based on comments from these two working groups, the draft was revised. It was then sent for further comments and criticisms to an expanded list of reviewers. Their comments were received by the end of August 1987.

In September 1987 the draft was revised, and subsequently sent to the Commission for approval. The Commission approved it by mail vote in October, and it was sent to the STG in mid-November.

APPENDIX B GLOSSARY OF TERMS

Accountability: Responsibility. Literally, being liable to give an account of one's conduct.

Acute: In health care, used to describe a condition that has a sudden onset, sharp rise, and short course. Acute diseases are generally completely resolved (compare **Chronic**).

Ambulatory care: Health care given to people who are not institutionalized.

Amyotrophic lateral sclerosis: A neurological disease leading to progressive muscular wasting with increased reflexes and irritability of the muscles.

Ancillary services or technology: Health care technology or services used directly to support basic clinical services, including diagnostic radiology, radiation therapy, clinical laboratory, and other special services. The term is most often used in connection with the hospital setting.

Antibiotic: A chemical substance (often produced by a micro-organism) that is administered to fight infections, usually bacterial infections, in humans or animals. The action of the antibiotic is to kill or inhibit the growth of the bacteria. Examples are pencillin, tetracycline, and erythromycin.

Apheresis: A procedure in which blood is separated into its basic components (red cells, white cells, platelets, and plasma), and one or more of these is selectively removed from the blood. The procedure is usually accomplished by removing venous whole blood from the body, separating the blood into cellular and noncellular (plasma) parts or fractions, and returning the cellular fraction to the patient.

Applied research: In the health care sector, an activity drawing on basic information to create solutions to problems in prevention, treatment, or cure of disease. Applied research seeks knowledge for the manipulation or control of vital processes.

Arteriosclerosis: A condition in which the arterial walls become thickened and hardened. The causes are multiple and complex, and often incompletely known. Also called 'hardening of the arteries'. See **Atherosclerosis.**

Arthritis: Inflammation of a joint.

Artifact: A physical object showing human workmanship or modification.

Artificial intelligence: A field of research and development involving computers. The attempt is to develop programs that can reason and solve problems at a higher level than is now possible.

Artificial organ: A machine or device that substitutes for an absent or inadequately functioning organ.

Asepsis: A condition in which living pathogenic organisms (germs) are absent.

Asthma: A disease marked by recurrent attacks of shortness of breath. Often the condition is caused by an underlying allery.

Atherosclerosis: A very common form of arteriosclerosis in which deposits of fibrous and cellular tissue, cholesterol, and fat accumulate in large and medium-sized arteries, impeding blood flow.

Basic research: An activity whose aim to understand vital processes. Basic research has as its goal to developing knowledge or understanding. Application of the knowledge occurs through applied research.

Biochemistry: Chemistry of living organisms and of the changes occurring therein.

Biofeedback: The technique of making unconscious or involuntary bodily processes (such as heartbeat or brain waves) perceptible to the senses in order to manipulate them by conscious mental control.

Biomaterials: Physical materials implanted into the human body. Biomaterials are used in joint implants, cardiac pacemakers, tooth implants, and so forth.

Biosensor: An instrument to detect and measure certain biological materials that is implanted in the human body.

Cadaveric: Having to do with a dead body.

Cancer: A tumor, the natural course of which is usually fatal. Cancers are divided into two broad categories, carcinoma and sarcoma.

Capitation: Per-head. Usually referring to a method of payment, such as to a general practitioner, when the provider of care is paid a fixed amount for each person, regardless of the number of services given.

Case management: Assessing of a person's needs and subsequent coordinating of the services provided.

Cataract: Loss of transparency of the lens of the eye.

Catheter: A hollow cylinder, usually of rubber or plastic, usually used to drain fluid, as from the urinary bladder.

Central nervous system: The brain and spinal cord. The nerves and ganglia outside of the central nervous system constitute the peripheral nervous system.

Chemotherapy: The use of specific chemical agents to arrest the progress of, or eradicate, disease in the body.

Chronic: Lingering, lasting, as opposed to acute. A term used to describe persistent or irreversible disease.

Chronic obstructive pulmonary disease: A disease of the lungs leading to continous shortness of breath.

Clinical trial: An experiment carried out for the purpose of evaluating the efficacy and safety of a health care technology. The nature of the control group is a critical issue in a clinical trial. See **Control group, Randomized clinical trial.**

Communicative disorder: A problem of communication, such as the inability to speak.

Congenital: Existing at birth.

Congenital abnormality: Any abnormality in structure or function, whether genetic or not, that has a prenatal origin (is present at birth). Congenital abnormalities can be genetic, chromosomal, or caused by endogenous or exogenous agents. Some prefer the term **Developmental disorder.**

Continuous ambulatory peritoneal dialysis: See **Peritoneal dialysis.**

Control group: In a randomized clinical trial, the group receiving no treatment or some treatment with which the group receiving experimental treatment is compared. The control treatment is generally a standard treatment, a placebo, or no treatment. Compare **Experimental group.**

Controlled clinical trial: See **Clinical trial.**

Coronary artery disease (coronary heart disease): Narrowing or blockage of the coronary arteries, which usually results in reduced blood flow to the heart muscle.

Cost-effectiveness analysis (CEA): An analytical technique that compares the costs of a project or of alternative projects to the resultant benefits, with costs and benefits/effectiveness expressed by different measures. Costs are usually expressed in dollars, but benefits/effectiveness are ordinarily expressed in terms such as 'lives saved,' 'disability avoided,' 'quality-adjusted life years saved,' or any other relevant objectives.

Cystic fibrosis: A hereditary disorder characterized by widespread dysfunction of glands. Problems in breathing and pulmonary infection are characteristic of the disease.

Cytotoxic: Destructive to cells.

Delivery system: See **Drug delivery system**.

Development: See **Applied research**. Also **Targeted development**.

Developmental disorder: See Congenital abnormality.

Diabetes mellitus: A disorder of carbohydrate (sugar) metabolism marked by elevated blood sugar due to faulty insulin production and abnormalities in different organs, including the eye, the kidney, and the peripheral nerves.

Diagnosis: The process of determining a person's illness from complaints and other information. See **Screening**.

Diagnostic kit: A simplified method of doing a diagnostic test that can be entirely packaged in one 'kit'. Such kits can be used anywhere, including in the home, and some of the tests can be performed relatively reliably by lay people.

Dialysis: The process of separating substancess in solution by the differences in their rates of diffusion through a semipermeable membrane. It is used especially in the treatment of end-stage renal (kidney) disease to remove otherwise poisonous substances that accumulate in the body. See **Peritoneal dialysis**.

Diffusion: See **Technology diffusion**.

Disability: A term used to denote the presence of one or more functional limitations. A person with a disability has a limited ability or an inability to perform one or more basic life functions (e.g., walking) at a level considered 'typical'. Compare to **Handicap**.

Drug delivery system: A method to improve the delivery of a drug within the body or to a certain site in the body. Delivery systems include pumps and implantable reservoirs.

Early warning system: A system with the purpose of alerting others, especially policy makers, to future developments of importance. An early warning system has been characterized as no more than a communication device between experts and policy makers.

Effectiveness: Same as efficacy (see below) except that it refers to '...average or actual conditions of use'.

Efficacy: The probability of benefit to individuals in a defined population from a medical technology applied for a given medical problem under ideal conditions of use.

Endocrine: Refers to a gland that furnishes an internal secretion. Examples are the pancreas and the gonads.

Endogenous: Developing or originating within the organism, or arising from causes within the organism.

End-stage renal disease (ESRD): Chronic renal failure that occurs when an individual's kidney is irreversibly damaged to such an extent that life cannot be sustained without treatment. Chronic renal dialysis, kidney transplant surgery, and continuous ambulatory peritoneal dialysis are forms of therapy.

Enteral therapy: The giving of nutrients by way of the intestine, usually by way of a tube. See **Parenteral therapy**.

Epilepsy: A chronic functional nervous disorder characterized by attacks of unconsciousness or convulsions or both.

Ergonomic: Confortable to use and functional. Ergonomics involves studying the posture of the body and effort expended by muscles to assure that the design of equipment is acceptable for human functioning.

Ethics: A generally shared set of felt duties, obligations, rights, ideas of justice, and of good and evil. The ethical system of a society is its collection of and operation on moral norms. Also used to refer to the study of such beliefs and values.

Experimental group: In a randomized clinical trial, the group receiving the treatment being evaluated for safety and efficacy. The experimental treatment may be a new technology, an existing technology applied to a new problem, or an accepted treatment about whose safety or efficacy there is doubt. Compare **Control group**.

Expert system: A computer program developed by an interdisciplinary group of medical experts for problem-solving. Expert systems are available to aid both medical diagnosis and medical treatment.

False negative: A negative test result in an individual who actually **does have** the disease or characteristic being tested for. The person is incorrectly diagnosed as not having a particular disease or characteristic.

False positive: A positive test result in an individual who does **not** have the disease or characteristic being tested for. I.e., the individual is incorrectly diagnosed as having a particular disease or characteristic.

First line care: Health care of immediate access. First line providers, such as general practitioners, are the first to be consulted in case of health problems. In the Netherlands, they control access to more specialized care.

Functional electrical stimulation: Stimulation of peripheral nerves by electric impulses to produce muscle contraction. It is used in cases of paralysis (especially from spinal cord damage) to produce muscular movement, generally in the arms or legs. Although systems are still primitive, some paralyzed patients have been able to walk up to 1 kilometer with functional electrical stimulation.

Futures research: Studies of the future. Futures research is not an attempt to predict the future, but analyzes the consequences of alternative decisions or actions.

Halfway technology: A term referring to health care technology that attempts to compensate for the incapacitating effects of certain diseases whose course one is unable to do much about. It is a technology designed to make up for disease or to postpone death. Transplants of organs and many cancer therapies are examples.

Handicap: Inability to perform one or more life functions (e.g., eating, conversing, working) at a 'typical' level, caused by the interaction of an individual's disability with the physical and social environments in which that person is functioning or expected to function. Compare to **Disability**.

Health care: The medical services provided by physicians, but also other services related to health, including rehabilitation, support for those with chronic illness or disability, and terminal care.

Health care technology: The drugs, devices, and medical and surgical procedures used in medical care, and the organizational and support systems within which such care is provided.

Health education: Methods of communication information and changing motivation concerning certain behaviors, with the aim of improving health.

Hemiplegia: Paralysis of one side of the body, usually caused by a stroke.

Hemodialysis: See **Dialysis**.

Hemophilia: A rare, hereditary bleeding disorder distinguished by a deficiency of one or more coagulation factors - e.g., Factor VIII (hemophilia A). Hemophilia is chiefly seen in males, and most often transmitted to offspring by asymptomatic females.

Holistic medicine: A type of medicine that actively attempts to deal with the person as a whole (e.g., rather than as an organism with a real or potential disease).

Home care: Care given in the home.

Home health care: The provision of health care services in the home rather than in an institutional setting or a provider's office.

Hormone: A chemical substance released into the circulatory system by glands belonging to the endocrine system, and that has a specific regulatory effect on another organ; functions regulated include metabolism, growth, and the development of secondary sex characteristics (such as breasts, facial hair).

Hospice: The palliative and supportive care for terminally ill patients and their families, either directly or on a consulting basis with the patients physician and/or district nurse.

Hypertension: High blood pressure.

Idiopathic: Denoting a primary disease without apparent extrinsic cause. The term is often used to mean 'of unknown cause'.

Implantable reservoir: A delivery system for a drug, implanted in the body, and releasing the drug over extended periods of time by diffusion or osmotic pressure.

Incidence: The frequency of new occurrences of disease within a defined time interval. Incidence rate is the number of new cases of specified disease over a specified period of time, usually 1 year, divided by the number of people in a population. Compare **Prevalence**.

Incontinence: Inability to prevent the discharge of excretions, especially of urine or feces.

Infection: The invasion and proliferation of any pathogenic organism in body tissues.

Information technology: The application of computers and telecommunication systems for the creation, storage, manipulation, and dissemination of information.

Innovation: A new device, product, or process introduced to practice for the first time. Innovations are valued for their capacity to improve the quality or decrease the costs of a given process or product. Also, something perceived to be new. In addition, innovation is widely used to refer to the process by which technological change occurs. See **Innovative process**.

Innovative process: The process by which innovations find their way into practice. The innovative process is seen as being made up of four stages: invention, development, entrepreneurship, and investment. See **Technological progress**.

Insulin: A substance produced by the pancreas and secreted into the blood with the function of enabling the organism to use sugar. Diabetes is characterized by a relative lack of insulin. Insulin is used to treat people with diabetes.

Intravenous: Into a vein.

Lesion: Structural change in a tissue or organ. See **Pathology**.

Managerial technology: Technology used to facilitate and support the provision of health care services, including administration, transportation, and communication, but not directly associated with patient care.

Man-machine interface: The relationship between people and their machines. This is now an active area of study and research. One aspect of this interface is ergonomics. Another is 'user-friendliness'.

Medical device: Any instrument, apparatus, or similar or related article that is intended to prevent, diagnose, mitigate, or treat disease or to affect the structure or function of the body.

Medicalization: A process by which normal or non-medical processes of life are seen as being disease-related and are brought into the health care system. It is often said that both birth and death have been 'medicalized' by modern society.

Medical technology: See **Health care technology.**

Metabolic: Referring to metabolism.

Metabolism: The sum of the chemical changes that make up the process of nutrition of the organism.

Microbiology: The science or study of microorganisms.

Migraine: Sick headache. Severe pain on one side of the head.

Molecule: The smallest possible quantity of a substance that can exist independently and still retain the properties of the substance of which it forms a part. It is formed by a combination of two or more atoms.

Monoclonal antibodies (MAbs): Antibodies derived from a single source or clone of cell. MAbs recognize only one type of antigen.

Morbidity: The condition of being diseased. The morbidity rate is the ratio of sick to well persons in a community.

Moribund: Dying. Close to death.

Mortality rate: The death rate, often made explicit for a particular characteristic, e.g., age, sex, or specific cause of death. A mortality rate contains three essential elements: 1) the number of people in a population group exposed to the risk of death; 2) a time factor; 3) the number of deaths occurring in the exposed population during a certain time period.

Myocardial infarction: Necrosis (death) of tissue in the myocardium (heart muscle) that results from insufficient blood supply to the heart.

Neonatal: Concerning the time immediately after birth.

Neurological: Referring to the nervous system (including the brain).

Osteomyelitis: Inflammation of the bone marrow.

Osteoporosis: A disease of bone marked by loss of calcium and resulting in softened or brittle bone, prone to fractures. It occurs frequently in elderly people, particularly women.

Palliative treatment: Treatment designed to relieve the symptoms of a disease or condition (e.g., to provide comfort or reduce pain), but not able to cure the disease or condition.

Parenteral nutrition: The supply of nutrients directly into the bloodstream (intravenously), circumventing the digestive tract.

Pathological: Relating to pathology. Morbid or diseased.

Pathology: The scientific study of the essential nature of disease and of the associated structural and functional changes in tissues and organs that are the result of disease. The field of pathology often deals with the diagnosis of disease. The term is also frequently used as a synonym for 'disease'.

Peer review: Review by equals. In quality assurance, used to refer to review by physicians of the quality of care given by other physicians

Peritoneal dialysis: A form of dialysis that occurs within the patient's body, rather than via an extracorporeal blood loop as in hemodialysis. A catheter is inserted into the abdomen and then dialysate is entered through the catheter into the peritoneal cavity. The fluid is allowed to remain for varying periods of time, during which dialysis occurs across the semi-permeable peritoneal membrane. Later, the dialysate is drained out through the catheter and discarded.

Pharmacology: The branch of science that is concerned with drugs (pharmaceuticals).

Physiology: The science which deals with living things, especially their normal vital processes.

Prevalence: The total number of cases of disease, infected persons, or persons with disabilities or some other condition, in existence in a particular area or population. The prevalence rate is the total number (prevalence) in relation to the size of the population. Compare **Incidence**.

Primary care: General health care, usually given on an ambulatory basis.

Procedure (medical or surgical): A health care technology involving any combination of drugs, devices, and provider skills and abilities. Appendectomy, for example, involves at least drugs (for anesthesia), monitoring devices, surgical devices, and the skilled actions of physicians, nurses, and support staff.

Prospective assessment: Assessment of a technology before it has been developed. Later in the life-cycle of the technology, data can be collected to make these assessments more realistic. A prospective assessment is, by definition, somewhat speculative. Nonetheless, it may be helpful for planning.

Prosthesis: An artificial substitute for a missing body part such as an arm or a leg.

Protocol: A formalized system describing medical decision-making. A state-of-the-art medical regimen.

Psychiatric: Relating to psychiatry, the diagnosis and treatment of diseases of the mind.

Pump: See **Implantable reservoir.**

Quality of care: The degree to which actions taken or not taken maximize the probability of beneficial health outcomes and minimize risk and or adverse outcomes, given the existing state of medical science and art.

Quality assessment: Measurement and evaluation of quality of care for individuals, groups, or populations.

Quality assurance: Refers to integrated programs that attempt to protect or raise quality of care by conducting assessments, taking action to correct problems found, and following up corrective interventions.

Quasi-experiment: A type of natural experiment that includes some aspects of an experiment. For example, it may be possible to develop a suitable control group for comparison in some naturally-occurring situations.

Radiologist: The medical specialist skilled in the diagnostic and therapeutic use of x-rays and other medical imaging equipment.

Random allocation: In a randomized clinical trial, allocation of individuals to treatment groups such that each individual has an equal probability of being assigned to any group.

Randomized clinical trial (RCT): An experiment designed to test the safety and efficacy of a medical technology in which people are randomly allocated to experimental or control groups, and outcomes are compared.

Rehabilitation: Technology with the aim of helping disabled people gain the highest possible level of functional ability.

Renal dialysis: See **Dialysis**.

Respirator: An apparatus for administering artificial respiration, especially for a prolonged period.

Respiratory: Relating to respiration (breathing).

Risk: A measure of the probability of an adverse or untoward outcome and the severity of the resultant harm to health of individuals in a defined population and associated with the use of a medical technology applied for a given medical problem under specified conditions of use.

Robot: An automatic apparatus or machine that performs functions ordinarily ascribed to human beings or operates with what appears to be (almost) human intelligence.

Robotics: The field involving the use of robots. With mechanical improvements and the incorporation of computers, robotics will have many potential health care applications in the future.

Safety: A judgment of the acceptability of risk in a specified situation. See also **Risk**.

Scenario: An account of the present situation of a society or a part thereof, of possible and desirable alternative future situations of that society, and of alternative sequences of events that from present circumstances could lead to such futures.

Screening: An attempt to detect high risk individuals or those with disorders that have not yet caused symptoms. Screening is followed by specific diagnostic procedures when positive. It is done for the purpose of intervention, i.e., to cure the disease or prevent problems associated with it.

Self-care: The unorganized health activities and health related decision-making by individuals, families, neighbours, friends, and so forth. It encompasses (at least) self-medication, self-treatment, social support in illness, and first aid.

Sensitivity: The true positive ratio. In referring to a diagnostic test, it is the extent to which abnormals are correctly classified.

Somatic: A term used to refer to body tissues apart from reproductive (germinal) tissues.

Specificity: The true negative ratio. In referring to a diagnostic test, it is the extent to which normals are correctly classified. Compare **sensitivity**.

Spinal cord: A portion of the central nervous system contained with the spinal canal in the back.

Stroke: Loss of function due to inadequate circulation of blood in the brain caused by sudden lesions in the blood vessels of the brain. This can be caused by heart failure, blockage of arteries or veins, or bleeding into the brain. This condition is often followed by permanent neurological damage.

Targeted development: The product-oriented development of a technology after basic and applied research have accumulated sufficient knowledge and technical means to make final realization of the envisaged produce rather likely.

Technological change: The process by which technology evolves over time.

Technological forecasting: The systematic investigation into the future development and diffusion of technology.

Technological progress: The introduction to practice of new and more useful means to serve human purposes.

Technology: The application of organized knowledge to practical ends.

Technology assessment: In general, a comprehensive form of policy research that examines the technical, economic, and social consequences of technological applications. It is especially concerned with unintended, indirect, or delayed social impacts. In health policy, however, the term more often is used to mean any form of policy analysis concerned with health care technology, especially the evaluation of efficacy and safety.

Technology diffusion: The diffusion or spread of a medical technology into the health care system. It is generally thought to involve in two phases: the initial phase in which decisions are made to adopt or reject the technology, and a subsequent phase in which decisions are made to use the technology.

Telecommunications: Communication at a distance through various means, including telegraph, telephone wire, or satellite. At present, a computer is often part of a communication system.

Telediagnostics: Diagnosis at a distance, using telecommunications.

Telemetry: The science or process of transmitting quantitative measurements (such as pressure, speed, or temperature) by radio to a distant site where the measurements are recorded.

Therapeutic technology: A technology with the aim to cure or relieve the symptoms of a disease or other medical condition.

Transplantation: With regard to human organs, the transplanting of a healthy organ (e.g., kidney, cornea, liver, and so on) from a donor, living or recently deceased, into a patient with absent or inadequate functioning of the equivalent organ.

Vaccine: A preparation of living, attenuated, or killed bacteria or viruses, fractions thereof, or synthesized antigens identical or similar to those found in the disease-causing organisms, administered to produce or increase immunity to a particular disease.

Ventilator: A machine for mechanical assistance to breathing.

APPENDIX C GLOSSARY OF ACRONYMS

AAW	Algemene Arbeidsongeschiktheids Wet
ABP	Algemeen Burgelijk Pensioenfonds
ADL	assistance in daily living
AWBZ	Algemene Wet Bijzondere Ziektekosten
CAPD	continuous ambulatory peritoneal dialysis
CSII	continuous subcutaneous insulin infusion
EURO	European Regional Office of the World Health Organization
EZ	Ministerie van Economische Zaken (Ministry of Economic Affairs)
GMD	gemeenschappelijke medische dienst
GP	general practitioner (huisarts)
GR	Gezondheidsraad (Health Council)
HPN	home parenteral nutrition
ICIDH	International Classification of Impairments, Disabilities, and Handicaps.
IRV	Instituut voor Revalidatie Vraagstukken (Hoensbroek)
MTD	Medisch Technologische Dienst (TNO)
NIG	Nationaal Informatiesysteem Gehandicapten
NIVEL	Nederlands Instituut voor Onderzoek van de Eerstelijnsgezondheidszorg
OTA	Office of Technology Assessment (U.S. Congress)
PACS	picture archiving and communications system
PERS	personal emergency responce system
PRIS	produkt informatie systeem
RIC	regionaal informatiecentrum
STG	Stuurgroep Toekomstscenario's Gezondheidszorg (The Steering Committee on Future Health Scenario's)
TENS	transcutaneous electrical nerve stimulation
TNO	Nederlandse Organisatie voor Toegepast Natuurwetenschappelijk Onderzoek (Netherlands Organization for Applied Scientific Research)
WHO	World Health Organization
WVC	Ministerie van Welzijn, Volksgezondheid en Cultuur (Ministry of Welfare, Public Health, and Cultural Affairs)

APPENDIX D REFERENCES

1. Ackerman LV, Burke MW. Artificial intelligence and image processing. Henry Ford Hospital Medical Journal 1985; 33: 142-145.

2. Alcock AJ, Hildes JA, Kaufert PA, Kaufert JM, Bickford J. Respiratory poliomyelitis: a follow-up study. Canadian Medical Association Journal 1984; 130: 1305-1310.

3. Amenta MO. Hospice in the United States, multiple models and varied programs. Nursing Clinics of North America 1985; 20: 269-279.

4. American College of Physicians, Health and Public Policy Committee. Home health care. Annals of Internal Medicine 1986; 105: 454-460.

5. Ancona-Berk VA, Chalmers TC. An analysis of the costs of ambulatory and inpatient care. American Journal of Public Health 1986; 76: 1102-1104.

6. Antoniskis A, Anderson BC, Van Volkinburg EJ. Feasibility of outpatient self-administration of parenteral antibiotics. Western Journal of Medicine 1978; 128: 203-206.

7. Arbogast JG, Dodrill WH. Diabetes home monitoring by telephone data entry. Primary Care 1985; 12: 573-579.

8. Avorn J, Langer E. Induced disability in nursing home patients: a controlled trial. Journal of the American Geriatrics Society 1982; 30: 397-400.

9. Bailey LB, Corda JJ. Diagnosis and treatment of nutrition disorders in older patients. Geriatrics 1984: 39: 67-71.

10. Balinsky W. Home health care: a comparative analysis of hospital-based and community-based agency patients. Home Health Care Services Quarterly 1984; 5: 45-60.

11. Banaszak EF, Travers H, Frazier M, et al. Home ventilator care. Respiratory Care 1981; 26: 1262-1268.

12. Banester HK, Driscoll RD, Greenwood RN, Cattell WR. Reuse of

haemodialysis equipment: convenience and cost effectiveness. British Medical Journal 1982; 285: 473-474.

13. Banta HD. Embracing or rejecting innovations: clinical diffusion of health care technology. In: Reiser SJ, Anbar M, eds. The machine at the bedside. London: Cambridge University Press, 1984: 65-92.

14. Banta HD, Behney CJ, Willems JS. Toward rational technology in medicine. New York: Springer Publishing Company, 1981.

15. Barhydt-Wezenaar N. Home care and hospice. In: Jonas S ed. Health care delivery in the United States. New York:Springer Publishing Company, 1986: 237-262.

16. Barker W. Geriatric rehabilitation: (missing) linch-pin in health services for the elderly. Presented at the meetings of the American Public Health Association, Anaheim, California, 11 November 1984.

17. Beek M, Van Eijk J, Rutten G. Huisartsen en specialisten over hun onderlinge taakafbakening. Medisch Contact, 1984; 39: 1247-1251.

18. Beek M, Van Eijk J, Rutten G. Verschuivingen van eerste naar tweede lijn: opvattingen van huisartsen en specialisten. Medisch Contact, 1985; 40: 299-302.

19. Beland F. Who are those most likely to be institutionalized, the elderly who receive comprehensive home care services or those who do not? Social Science and Medicine 1985; 20: 347-354.

20. van Bemmel JH. Man and computer in the hospital of tomorrow. Amsterdam: Department of Medical Informatics, Free University of Amsterdam, 1985.

21. Bell PM, Walshe K. Home blood glucose monitoring, impact on lifestyle and diabetes control. The Practitioner 1984; 228: 197-202.

22. Berkman L, Breslow L. Health and ways of living. New York: Oxford University Press, 1983.

23. Besteman A, Dresme, De Boom van Duin F. Eindverslag van het experiment 24-uurs zorgverlening te Tholen/St. Philipsland. Goes, Provinciale Vereniging van het Zeeuwse Kruis, 1985.

24. Birnbaum HG, Kidder D. What does hospice cost? American Journal of Public Health 1984; 74: 689-697.

25. Blackshear PJ. Implantable infusion pumps: clinical applications. Methods in Enzymology 1985; 112: 520-530.

26. Blanpain JE. The changing environment of health care. International Journal of Technology Assessment in Health Care 1985; 1: 271-277.

27. Blum BI. Artificial intelligence and medical informatics. Medical Informatics 1986; 11: 3-18.

28. Boerma WGW. Gezinsverzorging. In: Sluijs EM, Dopheide JP, Van der Zee J. (red.), 1985.

29. Boerma WGW. Preventieve zorg in gezondheidscentra en groepspraktijken. Utrecht, NIVEL, 1985.

30. Boerma WGW, Groenewegen PP. Werkgebieden in gezondheidscentra vergeleken: wijk- of praktijkgebonden werken door huisartsen, wijkverpleging en maatschappelijk werk. In: Vademecum Eerstelijnszorg, Alphen aan de Rijn, Samson, 1985.

31. Boerma WGW. Stervens- en rouwbegeleiding vanuit gezondheidscentra. Utrecht, Nederlands Huisartsen Instituut, 1982.

32. Bonnet PD, Ruderman AP. Health care systems and financing. In Reinke WA ed. Health planning, qualitative aspects and quantitative techniques. Baltimore, Maryland: The Johns Hopkins Press, 1972 :209-218.

33. Boots JMJ. Het werk van de huisarts: resultaten van een functie-analyse in 93 huisartspraktijke. Rijksuniversiteit Limburg, Maastricht, 1983.

34. Brakebill JI, Robb RA. Ivey MF, Christensen DB, Young JH, Scribner BH. Pharmacy department costs and patient charges associated with home parenteral nutrition program. American Journal of Hospital Pharmacology 1983; 40: 260-263.

35. Bremer Schulte M. Self-help in medical education. In Hatch S, Kickbusch I eds. Self-help and health in Europe. Copenhagen: World Health Organization, 1983: 77-89.

36. Bremer Schulte M, Pluym B, van Schendle G. Reintegration with duos: a self-care program following myocardial infarction. Patient Education and Counseling 1986; 8: 233-244.

37. Brodie DC, Smith WE. Implications of new technology for pharmacy education and practice. American Journal of Hospital Pharmacy 1985; 42: 81-95.

38. Brooks CH, Smyth-Staruch K. Hospice home care cost savings to third-party insurers. Medical Care 1984; 22: 691-703.

39. Brown AK, Anderson U, Burch J, Nelson P. Home recording of arrhythmias by patients using a portable electrocardiograph. Journal of the Royal College of Physicians of London 1982; 16: 175-177.

40. Brown MM, Cornwell J, Kelleher E, Weist JK. Learned helplessness among the institutionalized elderly: a pilot study. Issues in Mental Health Nursing 1981; 3: 293-303.

41. Burr BH, Guyer B, Todres ID et al. Home care for children on respirators. New England Journal of Medicine 1983; 209: 1319-1323.

42. Burr ML. Nutritional epidemiology. Progress in Food and Nutrition Science 1985; 9: 149-183.

43. Cabin B. Cost-effectiveness of pediatric home care. Caring 1985; 4: 48-51.

44. Care for Life. Life sustaining technologies and the elderly: prolonged mechanical ventilation, data on utilization and cost. Paper Prepared for the Office of Technology Assessment, U.S. Congress, Washington DC, October 1985.

45. Carney K. An economic perspective on hospice. In: Musacchio R, Hough D, eds. Socioeconomic issues of health 1981. Chicago: American Medical Association, 1981: 93-108.

46. Centraal Begeleidingsorgaan voor de Intercollegiale Toetsing (CBO). Consensus osteoporosis. Resultaat van een consensus-bijeenkomst op 31 mei en 1 juni 1985 te Rotterdam.

47. Centraal Bureau voor de Statistiek. Overledenen naar doodsoorzaak, leeftijd en geslacht in het jaar 1980. CBS, Voorburg, 1981.

48. de Charro F, Banta D. Transplant policy in the Netherlands. International Journal of Technology Assessment in Health Care 1986; 2: 533-544.

49. Check WA. New drugs and drug-delivery systems in the year 2000. American Journal of Hospital Pharmacy 1984; 41: 1536-1547.

50. Commissie Structuur en Financiering Gezondheidszorg. Bereidheid tot verandering. 's-Gravenhage: Distributiecentrum Overheidspublikaties, 1987.

51. Committee on Science, Engineering, and Public Policy of the National Academy of Sciences, the National Academy of Engineering, and the Institute of Medicine. Outlook of science and technology: the next five years. Volume III. Washington, D.C.: National Academy Press, 1982.

52. US Congress, Senate, Committee on Finance. End-stage renal disease (ESRD) program under Medicare. Committee Print No. 97-9, 97th Congress, 1st Session, 1981.

53. Cooper BA, Gowland C, McIntosh J. The use of color in the environment of the elderly to enhance function. Clinics in Geriatric Medicine, 1986; 2: 151-163.

54. Copeland EM. The implications of industry moving into the field of home parenteral nutrition. Journal of Parenteral and Enteral Nutrition 1985; 9: 1-2.

55. Cottier C. Julius S, Gajendragadkar SV, Schork MA. Usefulness of home BP determination in treating borderline hypertension. Journal of the American Medical Association 1982; 248: 555-558.

56. Creek van de L. A home care hospice profile: description, evaluation and cost analysis. Journal of Family Practice 1982; 14: 53-58.

57. Cummings RO, Eisenberg MS, Bergner L, Hallstrom A, Hearne T, Murray JA. Automatic external defibrillation: evaluations of its role in the home and in emergency medical services. Annals of Emergency Medicine 1984; 13: 796-801.

58. Curtiss FR. Reimbursement dilemma regarding home health-care products and services. American Journal of Hospital Pharmacology 1984; 41: 1548-1557.

59. Delano BG, Lundin Ap, Friedman EA. Successful home hemodialysis in purportedly unacceptable patients. Nephron 1982; 31: 191-193.

60. Dinkel R. Parenteral nutrition in different settings: results of an economic study. International Journal of Technology Assessment in Health Care 1985; 1: 335-341.

61. Doherty H, Hicks N. Cost-effectiveness analysis and alternative health care programs for the elderly. Health Services Research 1977; 12: 190-203.

62. Donn S. Cost effectiveness of home management of bronchopulmonary dysplasia (letter). Pediatrics 1982; 70: 330-331.

63. Dopheide JP. Verwijzingen door de huisarts: enkele determinanten van het verwijscijfer van solo-huisartsen op het verstedelijkt platteland en in forensengemeenten. Gezondheid en Samenleving, 1982; 3: 141-151.

64. Doshi ML. Accuracy of consumer performed in-home tests for early pregnancy detection. American Journal of Public Health 1986; 76: 512-514.

65. Doty P. Family care of the elderly: the role of public policy. The Milbank Quarterly 1986; 64: 34-75.

66. Dowie R. Deployment of resources in treatment of end stage renal failure in England and Wales. British Medical Journal 1984; 31: 988-991.

67. Dubos R. Man adapting. New Haven, Connecticut: Yale University Press, 1965, 1980.

68. Dunkin LJ. Home ventilatory assistance. Anaesthesia 1983; 3811: 644-649.

69. Dzierba SH, Mirtallo JM, Grauer DW, Schneider PJ, Latiolais CJ, Fabri PJ. Fiscal and clinical evaluation of home parenteral nutrition. American Journal of Hospital Pharmacology 1984; 41: 285-291.

70. ECRI. Cochlear implants for profound deafness. Issues in health care technology. New technology briefs/5/C.1, 1983.

71. ECRI. Implantable drug infusion pumps. Issues in health care technology. New technology briefs/5.I.4, 1982.

72. ECRI. Insulin delivery devices. Issues in health care technology. New Technology Briefs/5.I.2. 1981.

73. ECRI. The Medicare dialysis program. Issues in health care technology. Ethics and Social Policy/2.2. 1982.

74. ECRI. New opportunities in high-technology home care. Issues in health care technology. Management/4.18. 1985.

75. ECRI. Outpatient surgery: its perils and prospects. Health technology 1987; 1: 91-98.

76. ECRI. Personal emergency response systems (PERSs). Issues in health care technology. New technology briefs/5.P.10, 1986.

77. ECRI. Robots: future additions to hospital staff. Issues in health care technology. Technology and People/18.7, 1986.

78. ECRI. Treatment of diabetes: a new technology, a new opportunity for hospitals. Issues in health care technology. Management/4.2. 1982.

79. Elliott GR, Eisdorfer C, eds. Stress and human health, analysis and implications of research. New York: Springer Publishing Company, 1982.

80. Elster J. Explaining technical change. Studies in rationality and social change. London: Cambridge University Press, 1983.

81. Enright M, Jonas S. Hospitals. In Jonas S. Health care delivery in the United States. New York: Springer Publishing Company, 1981: 169-217.

82. Eron LJ. Intravenous antibiotic administration in outpatient settings. Infectious DIsease 1984; 41: 285-291.

83. Eschbach JW, Swymour M, Potts A, Clark M, Blagg CR. A hemodialysis orientation unit. Nephron 1983; 33: 106-110.

84. Fall M, Carlsson CA. Current progress in the treatment of urinary dysfunctions. International Journal of Technology Assessment in Health Care 1985; 1: 397-417.

85. Feldman J, Tuteur PG. Mechanical ventilation: from hospital intensive care to home. Heart & Lung 1982; 11: 162-165.

86. Fischer DA, Prentice WS. Feasibility of home care for certain respiratory-dependent restrictive or obstructive lung disease patients. Chest 1982; 82: 739-743.

87. Flasterstein F, Klocke RA. Outpatient oxygen therapy. Primary CAre 1982; 9: 127-134.

88. Foets M, Van der Velden J, Van der Zee J. Een Nationale Studie van ziekten en verrichtingen in de huisartspraktijk; projectvoorstel. NIVEL, Utrecht, 1986.

89. Gemeenschappelijke Medische Dienst. Jaarverslag 1985. GMD, Amsterdam, 1986.

90. Gemeenschappelijke Medische Dienst. Statistische Informatie 1985. GMD, Amsterdam, 1986

91. George CR. Feasibility of universal home haemodialysis with simplified techniques. Lancet 1983; 2: 895-897.

92. Gershuny JI. Reflections on home-based health services and the future of the service sector. International Journal of Technology Assessment in Health Care 1985; 1: 365-369.

93. Gezondheidsraad. Advies inzake dialyse en niertransplantatie. The Hague, The Netherlands. 1986.

94. Gezondheidsraad. Advies inzake kwaliteitsbeheer medische hulpmiddelen. The Hague, The Netherlands. 19 August 1985.

95. Gezondheidsraad. Kwaliteitsbeheer medische hulpmiddelen. The Hague, The Netherlands. 19 August 1985.

96. Gezondheidsraad. Medische biotechnologie. The Hague, The Netherlands. 24 October 1985.

97. Gezondheidsraad. Pancreastransplantatie. The Hague, The Netherlands. 30 October 1985.

98. Gibbins FJ, Lee M, Davison PR, O'Sullivan P, Huthinson M, Murphy DR, UGwu CN. Augmented home nursing as an alternative to hospital care for chronic elderly invalids. British Medical Journal of Clinical Research 1982; 284: 330-333.

99. Goldberg AI. The Illinois plan. In Report of the Surgeon General's Workshop on Children with Handicaps and Their Families. (DHHS Pub.

No. PHS-83-50194). Washington DC: US Department of Health and Human Services, 1983.

100. Goldberg AI, Faure EAM. Home care for life-supported persons in England, the responaut program. Chest 1986; 6: 910-914.

101. Goldberg AI, Faure EA, Vaughn CJ, et al. Home care for life-supported persons: an approach to program development. Journal of Pediatrics 1984; 104: 785-795.

102. Gotay CC. Models of terminal care: a review of the research literature. Clinical and Investigative Medicine 1983; 6: 131-141.

103. Grant L, Swain I. Meeting report: functional electrical stimulation. Journal of Medical Engineering & Technology 1985; 9: 129-131.

104. Greer AL. Deus ex machina: physicians in the adoption of hospital medical technology (manuscript). Milwaukee: Urban Research Center, The University of Wisconsin-Milwaukee, 1981.

105. Groenewegen PP. Locatiekeuze en huisartsendichtheid: een verklaring van regionale verschillen en veranderingen. NIVEL, Utrecht, 1985.

106. Groenewegen PP, Kerssens JJ, Curfs EChr. Physiotherapy and the care for disabled and chronically ill people in the community. Paper presented at the WHO consultation on 'care of disabled people in the community', Edinburg, June 1986.

107. Groth-Juncker A, McCusker J. Where do elderly patients prefer to die? Place of death and patient characteristics of 100 elderly patients under the care of a home health care team. Journal of the American Geriatric Society 1983; 31: 457-461.

108. Gunning-Schepers L, Leroy X, De Wals P. Home care as an alternative to hospitalization: a case study in Belgium. Social Science and Medicine 1984; 18: 531-537.

109. Haber PAL. Technology in aging. The Gerontologist 1986; 26: 350-357.

110. Haga T. A study of long-term oxygen therapy in Japan and other Asian countries. Respiratory Care 1983; 28: 922-925.

111. Hamers RTJ, Boerma WGW. Het dienstenaanbod van huisartsen in verschillende praktijkvormen. NIVEL, Utrecht, 1985.

112. Hammond J. Home health care cost effectiveness: an overview of the literature. Public Health Reports 1979; 94: 305-311.

113. Harper AE. Coronary heart disease - an epidemic related to diet? The American Journal of Clinical Nutrition 1983; 37: 669-681.

114. Harris LF, Buckle TF, Coffey Fl. Intravenous antibiotics at home. Southern Medical Journal 1986; 79: 193-196.

115. Harris WL, McAllister JC. Microcomputer applications for home health-care services. American Journal of Hospital Pharmacy 1985; 42: 2702-2706.

116. Hazard MP. Home health care: on the increase. Journal of MAC 1986; 75: 275-277.

117. Hedrick SC, Inui TS. The effectiveness and cost of home care: an information synthesis. Health Services Research 1986; 20: 851-880.

118. Heesters JP. De honorering van de Nederlandse huisarts als vrijberoeps beoefenaar en de relatie met de goodwill problematiek. Katholieke Hogeschool, Tilburg, 1983.

119. Hermesse J. Cost-effective health technology at home as an avenue for reducing national health expenditures: a view from government. International Journal of Technology Assessment in Health Care 1985; 1: 289-300.

120. Hickam DH, Shortliffe EH, Bischoff MB, Scott AC, Jacobs CD. The treatment advice of a computer-based cancer chemotherapy protocol advisor. Annals of Internal Medicine 1985; 103: 928-936.

121. Hingstman L. Cijfers uit de registratie van beroepen in de eerstelijns gezondheidszorg. NIVEL, Utrecht, 1985.

122. Holtzman NA. The application of recombinant DNA technology to genetic testing: promise and peril. (Manuscript of book, in press)

123. Hopper SV, Miller JP, Birge C, Swift J. A randomized study of the impact of home health aides on diabetic control and utilization patterns. American Journal of Public Health 1984; 74: 600-602.

124. Horl J, Rosenmayr L. Assistance to the elderly as a common task of the family and social service organization. Archives of Gerontology and Geriatrics 1982; 1: 75-95.

125. Howard L, Michalek AV. Home parenteral nutrition. Annual Reviews of Nutrition 1984; 4: 69-99.

126. Innovatie Hulpmiddelen Gehandicapten. 2e herziening meerjarenplan. Maarssen, 1986.

127. Institute of Medicine. Health and behavior. Washington, DC: National Academy Press, 1982.

128. Institute of Medicine. Health, behavior, and aging. Washington, DC: National Academy Press, 1981.

129. Jackson BN. Home health care and the elderly in the 1980s. The American Journal of Occupational Therapy 1984; 38: 717-720.

130. Jackson B, Jensen J. Home care leads rising trend of new services. Modern Healthcare December 1984: 34-35.

131. Joyeux H, Gouttebel MC, Rodier F, Lacour B, Salassol C. Home total parenteral nutrition in France. International Journal of Technology Assessment in Health Care 1985; 1: 325-333.

132. Kahn L. Ventilator-dependent children heading home. Hospitals 1984; 58: 54-55.

133. Kane RL, Wales J, Bernstein L, Leibowitz A, Kaplan S. A randomized controlled trial of hospice care. Lancet 1984; 1: 890-894.

134. Kaplan BH, Cassel JC, Gork S. Social support and health. Medical Care 1977; 15: 47-58.

135. Kelsay Jl, Hochberg MC. Epidemiology and prevention of musculoskeletal disorders. In Last JM ed. Public health and preventive medicine. Norwalk, Connecticut: Appleton-Century-Crofts, 1986: 1277-1295.

136. Kennie DC. Good health care for the aged. Journal of the American Medical Association 1983; 249: 770-773.

137. Kerkstra A, Verhaak PFM. Wijkverpleging. In: Sluijs EM, Dopheide JP, Van der Zee J. (red.), 1985.

138. Kersten TJJMT. Samenwerking tussen maatschappelijk werk en gezondheidszorg in de eerste lijn. NIVEL, Utrecht, 1985a, 1985.

139. Kersten TJJMT. Algemeen maatschappelijk werk. In: Sluijs EM, Dopheide JP, Van der Zee J. (red.), 1985b, 1985.

140. Kickbusch I, Hatch S. Introduction: a reorientation of health care? In Hatch S, Kickbusch I eds. Self-help and health in Europe. Copenhagen: World Health Organization, 1983: 1-9.

141. Kind AC, Williams DN, Persons G, Gibson JR. Intravenous antibiotic therapy at home. Archives of Internal Medicine 1979; 139: 413-415.

142. Klarman HE, Francis JO, Rosenthal GD. Cost effectiveness analysis applied to the treatment of chronic renal disease. Medical Care 1968; VI: 48-

143. Koren MJ. Home care - who cares? New England Journal of Medicine 1986; 314: 917-920.

144. Krijgsman AR. Georganiseerde nazorg in Nederland: een inventarisatie van wijkverpleegkundige nazorg. NIVEL, Utrecht, 1986.

145. Lakshmanan M, Mion LC, Frengley JD. Effective low dose tricyclic antidepressant treatment for depressed geriatric rehabilitation patients. A double-blind study. Journal of the American Geriatrics Society 1986; 34: 421-426.

146. Lameire NH. Experience with CAPD as home dialysis. International Journal of Technology Assessment in Health Care 1985; 1: 305-313.

147. Last JM. Scope and methods of prevention. In Last JM ed. Public health and preventive medicine. Norwalk, Connecticut: Appleton-Century-Crofts, 1986: 3-7.

148. Lee GB. Development of a home health care management program in Los Angeles County. California Children Services, Department of Health Services, County of Los Angeles, October 31, 1983.

149. Leemeijer M, Suurmeijer ThPBM, van den Heuvel WJA. Thuiszorg door 24-uurs kruiszorg: verslag van een evaluatieonderzoek naar 7x24 uurszorgverlening bij de wijkverlening in Friesland. Groningen: vakgroep Medische Sociologie Rijksuniversiteit Groningen 1986.

150. van der Lei J. Ervaringen met medische expertsystemen. Vakgroep Medische Informatica, Vrije Universiteit Amsterdam (manuscript), June 1986.

151. Lerner H, Giner J, Soeldner JS, Colton CK. An implantable electrochemical glucose sensor. Annals of the New York Academy of Sciences 1984; 428: 263-278.

152. Levine RE. The cultural aspects of home care delivery. The American Journal of Occupational Therapy 1984; 38: 734-738.

153. Liang MH, Gall V, Partridge A, Eaton H. Management of functional disability in homebound patients. Journal of Family Practice 1983; 17: 429-435.

154. Liem PH, Chernoff R, Carter WJ. Geriatric rehabilitation unit: a 3-year outcome evaluation. Journal of Gerontology 1986; 41: 44-50.

155. Loucks VR. Home health care: a perspective from industry. International Journal of Technology Assessment in Health Care 1985; 1: 301-304.

156. Lowson KV, Drummond MF, Bishop JM. Costing new services: long-term domiciliary oxygen therapy. Lancet 1981; 1: 1146-1149.

157. Ludbrook A. The economics of home care for the treatment of end-stage renal failure. International Journal of Technology Assessment in Health Care 1985; 1: 315-324.

158. McKay AB. Computers in home health care: present and future impact. American Pharmacy 1985; NS25: 48-51.

159. McKinlay JB. Social network influences on morbid episodes and the career of help seeking. In Eisenberg L, Kleinman A eds. The Relevance of social science for medicine. Dordrecht, The Netherlands: D. Reidel Publishing Company 1980: 77-107.

160. McNerney WJ. The rationale for siting advanced health technologies at home. International Journal of Technology Assessment in Health Care 1985; 1: 279-288.

161. Mann NP, Noronha JI, Johnston DI. A prospective study to evaluate the benefits of long-term self-monitoring of blood glucose in diabetic children. Diabetes Care 1984; 7: 322-326.

162. Ministerie van Welzijn, Volksgezondheid en Cultuur. Nota Eerstelijnszorg. Staatsuitgeverij, s'-Gravenhage, 1983.

163. Ministerie van Welzijn, Volksgezondheid en Cultuur. Nota Volksgezondheid bij beperkte middelen. Staatsuitgeverij, s'-Gravenhage, 1983.

164. Ministerie van Welzijn, Volksgezondheid en Cultuur. Nota Flankerend Bejaardenbeleid. Staatsuitgeverij, s'-Gravenhage, 1983.

165. Ministerie van Welzijn, Volksgezondheid en Milieuhygiene. Nota Patientenbeleid. Staatsuitgeverij, s'-Gravenhage, 1981.

166. Ministerie van Welzijn, Volksgezondheid en Milieuhygiene. Nota 2000 over de ontwikkeling van het gezondheidsbeleid. Rijswijk, 1986.

167. Mohan R, Caley R. Standardization of therapy machine interface for treatment monitoring. International Journal of Radiation Oncology Biology and Physics 1983; 9: 1225-1229.

168. Munro HN. Nutriment needs and nutritional status in relation to aging. Drug-Nutrient Interactions 1985; 4: 55-74.

169. Munro HN. Nutrition and the elderly: a general overview. Journal of the American College of Nutrition 1984; 3: 341-350.

170. Mutchie KD, Mackay MW, Marsh C. Juluson D. Pharmacist monitoring of parenteral nutrition: clinical and cost effectiveness. American Journal of Hospital Pharmacology 1979; 36: 785-787.

171. Nanny G, Stella G, et al. Home total parenteral nutrition. Minerva Chirurgica 1984; 39: 311-317.

172. National Institute of Allergy and Infectious Diseases. Status of vaccines targeted for accelerated development. Presented at Congressional Hearings on Biotechnology: Vaccine Development. Washington, DC: US Government Printing Office, 1985.

173. National Institutes of Health. Infantile apnea & home monitoring. Consensus Development Conference

174. Nationale Kruisvereniging. Kruiswerk in beeld; verantwoording 1981-1985. Meerjarenraming 1987-1990. Kruiswerk. Bunnik, 1985.

175. Nelson EC, McHugo G, Schnurr P, Devito C, Roberts E, Simmons J, Zubkoff W. Medical self-care education for elders: a controlled trial to evaluate impact. American Journal of Public Health 1984; 74: 1357-1362.

176. Nelson RJ. Hospice: an alternative solution to the problem of caring for the dying patient. Colloquy 1974: 22.

177. Nissel M, Bonnerjea L. Family care of the handicapped elderly: who pays? London: Policy Studies Institute, 1982.

178. Office of Technology Assessment. Assistive devices for severe speech impairments. Health technology case study 26. Washington DC: US Government Printing Office, 1983.

179. Office of Technology Assessment. Commercial biotechnology: an international analysis. Washington, DC: US Government Printing Office, 1984.

180. Office of Technology Assessment. The contact lens industry: structure, competition, and public policy. Health Technology Case Study 31. Washington DC: US Government Printing Office, 1984.

181. Office of Technology Assessment. Federal policies and the medical devices industry. Washington, DC: U.S. Government Printing Office, 1984.

182. Office of Technology Assessment. Technologies for managing urinary incontinence. Washington, DC: US Government Printing Office, 1985.

183. Office of Technology Assessment. Technology and handicapped people. Washington, DC: US Government Printing Office, 1982.

184. Office of Technology Assessment. Technology and aging in America. Washington, DC: US Government Printing Office, 1985.

185. Office of Technology Assessment. Technology-dependent children: hospital v. home care. Washington DC: US Government Printing Office, 1987.

186. Orleans M, Orleans P. High and low technology: sustaining life at home. International Journal of Technology Assessment in Health Care 1985; 1: 353-363.

187. Osterweis M, Solomon F, Green M, eds. Bereavement, reactions,

consequences, and care. Washington, DC: National Academy Press, 1984.

188. Oxygen in the home. Drug and Therapeutics Bulletin 1982; 30: 65-67.

189. Perry B, Lierman C. Hospital based pediatric home care: review of the issue and a case example. Report Submitted to the Robert Wood Johnson Foundation, June 28, 1985.

190. Petranyi G, Petranyi M, Scobie IN, Sonksen PH, Crane R, Roberts J, Menzies IS. Quality control of home monitoring of blood glucose concentrations. British Medical Journal 1984; 288: 757.

191. Poulshock SW, Deimling GT. Families caring for elders in residence: issues in the measurement of burden. Journal of Gerontology 1984; 39: 230-239.

192. Puska P, Tuomilehto J, Salonen J, Nissinen A, Virtamo J, Bjorkqvist S, Koskela K, Neittaanmaki L, Takalo T, Kottke T, Maki J, Sipila P, Varvikko KP. Community control of cardiovascular disease, The North Karelia Project. Copenhagen: The World Health Organization, Regional Office for Europe, 1981.

193. van Ree JW, Van Gerwen W, Van den Hoogen H. Interventie bij verhoogd risico op hart- en vaatziekten: resultaten op langere termijn van interventie bij hypercholesterolemie, adipositas en roken. Huisarts en Wetenschap, 1985; 28: 21-24.

194. van Ree JW, Van Gerwen W, Van den Hoogen H. Interventie bij een verhoogd risico op hart- en vaatziekten: resultaten op langere termijn bij de behandeling van hypertensie. Huisarts en Wetenschap, 1985; 28: 53-58.

195. Rehm SJ, Weinstein AJ. Home intravenous antibiotic therapy: a team approach. Annals of Internal Medicine 1983; 99: 388-392.

196. Roberts SD, Maxwell DR., Gross TL. Cost-effective care of end-stage renal disease: a billion dollar question. Annals of Internal Medicine 1980; 92: 243-248.

197. Robertson D. Alternative methods of health care delivery for Canada's aging population. Presented to the Colloguium on Aging with Limited Health Resources, Winnipeg, Canada, 5-6 May 1986.

198. Roolvink EGJJ. Huisarts en surveillance. Medisch Contact, 1985; 40: 609-610.

199. Rowe JW. Health care of the elderly. The New England Journal of Medicine 1985; 312: 827-835.

200. Rubenstein LZ. Effectiveness of a geriatric evaluation unit. A randomized clinical trial. The New England Journal of Medicine 1984; 311: 1664-1670.

201. Ruchlin HS, Morris JN. Pennsylvania's domiciliary care experiment: II. Cost-benefit implications. American Journal of Public Health 1983; 73: 654-660.

202. Russell LB. Is prevention better than cure? Washington, DC: The Brookings Institution, 1986.

203. Russell LB. Technology in hospitals: medical advances and their diffusion. Washington, DC: The Brookings Institutions, 1979.

204. Rutten G, Van Eijk J, Beek M. Huisarts, huidarts of patient. Medisch Contact, 1985; 40: 325-326.

205. Rutten G, Van Eijk J, Beek M. Kleine chirurgie: door wie? Medisch Contact, 1985; 40: 367-368.

206. Rutten G, Van Eijk J, Beek M. Controles bij diabetes mellitus: een peilend onderzoek naar opvattingen van huisartsen en internisten. Medisch Contact, 1985; 40: 389-390.

207. Rutten G, Van Eijk J, Beek M. Huisartsen en gynaecologen over taakafbakening en zelfzorg. Medisch Contact, 1985; 40: 432-434.

208. Rutten G, Van Eijk J, Beek M. Chronische bronchitus: opvattingen van huisartsen en longartsen over hun onderlinge taak en rol van de patient. Medisch Contact 1985; 40: 457-458.

209. Scenario Commission on Future Health Care Technology. Anticipating and assessing health care technology, volume 1, general considerations and policy conclusions. Dordrecht, The Netherlands: Martinus Nijhoff Publishers, 1987.

210. Schersten T. Home diagnostic tests. International Journal of Technology Assessment in Health Care 1985; 1: 441-442.

211. Schlag P. Continuous cancer chemotherapy: rationale and prerequisites for treatment at home. International Journal of Technology Assessment in Health Care 1985; 1: 343-351.

212. Sherman M, McLean D, Zorn E, et al. Home care for ventilator-dependent patients: a rational option (abstract). Respiratory Care 1982; 27: 1252.

213. Shonkoff JP. Social support and the development of vulnerable children. American Journal of Public Health 1984; 74: 310-312.

214. Siperstein MD. Diabetic microangiopathy and the control of blood glucose. New England Journal of Medicine 1983; 309: 1577-1579.

215. Sivak ED, Cordasco EM, Gipson WT, et al. Pulmonary mechanical ventilation at home: a reasonable and less expensive alternative. Respiratory Care 1983; 28: 42-49.

216. Sivak ED. Gipson WT, Hanson MR. Long-term management of respiratory failure in amyotrophic lateral sclerosis. Annals of Neurology 1982; 12: 18-23.

217. Skellie FA, Mobley GM, COan RE. Cost-effectiveness of community-based long-term care: current findings of Georgia's alternative health services project. American Journal of Public Health 1982; 72: 353-358.

218. Skyler JS. Complications of diabetes mellitus: relationship to metabolic dysfunction. Diabetes Care 1979; 1: 499-509.

219. Sluijs EM. Huisarts. In: Sluijs EM, Dopheide JP, Van der Zee J. (red.) 1985.

220. Sluijs EM, Dopheide JP, Van der Zee J. (red.). Overzichtsstudie onderzoek eerstelijn; stand van het wetenschappelijk onderzoek in en over de eerstelijns gezondheidszorg en haar raakvlakken. NIVEL, Utrecht, 1985.

221. Smith WE. Ethical, eonomic, and professional issues in home health care. American Journal of Hospital Pharmacy 1986; 43: 695-698.

222. van Sonderen FLP, Suurmeijer ThPBM, van den Heuvel WJA. Op maat gemeten; verslag van een onderzoek naar 7 x 24 uurs hulp bij de gezinsverzorging in Velp. Groningen: Vakgroep Medische Sociologie, 1985.

223. Spencer H, Kramer L. Factors contributing to osteoporosis. The American Journal of Clinical Nutrition 1983; 116: 316-319.

224. Splaingard ML, Splaingard D. Home care of the ventilator-dependent child: realities and limitations. Pride Institute Journal of Long Term Home Health Care 1986; 5: 15-20.

225. Spyker DA, Stier DM, O'Dell RW, Anne A, Edlich RF. A user-oriented information system for emergency medicine. Comprehensive Therapy 1984; 10: 42-47.

226. Stamler J. Nutrition-related risk factors for the atherosclerotic diseases - present status. Progress in Biochemical Pharmacology 1983; 19: 245-308.

227. Stange P, Sumner A. Predicting treatment costs and life expectancy for end-stage renal disease. New England Journal of Medicine 1978; 298: 372-378.

228. Steel K, Markson E, Crescenzi C, Hoffman S, Bissonnette A. An analysis of types and costs of health care services provided to an elderly inner-city population. Medical Care 1982; 20: 1090-1100.

229. Steinfeld E, Hiatt L. Multiple disability through the lifespan. Washington, DC: ATBCB, 1983: 1.3-1.7.

230. Steinhauer MJ. Occupational therapy and home health care. The American Journal of Occupational Therapy 1984; 38: 715-716.

231. Stell K, Markson E, Crescenzi C, Hoffman S, Bissonnette A. An analysis of types and costs of health care services provided to an elderly inner-city population. Medical Care 1982; 20: 1909-1100.

232. Stichting Toekomstbeeld der Techniek no. 42: "Techniek voor ouderen". Den Haag.

233. Stiver HG, Trosky SK, Cote DD, Oruck JL. Self-administration of intravenous antibiotics: an efficient, cost-effective home care program. Canadian Medical Association Journal 1982; 127: 207-211.

234. Stuurgroep Toekomstscenario's Gezondheidszorg (STG). Anticipating and assessing health care technology. Dordrecht: Martinus Nijhoff Publishers, 1987.

235. Stuurgroep Toekomstscenario's Gezondheidszorg (STG). Het hart van de toekomst, de toekomst van het hart. Scenario's over hart en vaatziekten 1985-2010. The Hague, 1986.

236. Stuurgroep Toekomstscenario's Gezondheidszorg (STG). Ouder worden in de toekomst. Scenario's over gezondheid en vergrijzing 1984-2000. The Hague, 1984.

237. Stuurgroep Toekomstscenario's Gezondheidszorg (STG). Lifestyles and health. The Hague, 1987.

238. Stuurgroep Toekomstscenario's Gezondheidszorg (STG). Kanker in Nederland. Rijswijk, 1987.

239. Swinkels MAA, Dopheide JP. Vervagende grenzen tussen eerste en tweede lijn: de casus Hoogeveen. Medisch Contact 1983; 38: 512-514.

240. Talonen P, Malmivuo J, Hakkinen V, Frey H. Functional electrical simulation in neurological disorders of lower extremities. Acta Neurologica Scandinavica 1984; 69: 401-402.

241. Taylor CE. Stages of the planning process. In Reinke WA ed. Health planning, qualitative aspects and quantitative techniques. Baltimore, Maryland: The Johns Hopkins Press, 1972: 20-34.

242. Turk R, Obreza P. Functional electrical stimulation as an orthotic means for the rehabilitation of paraplegic patients. Paraplegia 1985; 23: 344-348.

243. Vereniging van Revalidatiecentra in Nederland. Revalidatie intra- en extramuraal; discussienota. VRIN, Utrecht, 1985.

244. Verhaak PFM. Interpretatie en behandeling van psycho-sociale klachten in de huisartspraktijk: een onderzoek naar verschillen tussen huisartsen. NIVEL, Utrecht, 1986.

245. Verhaak PFM, Busschbach JT, Kortenhoeven D. Behoefte aan wijkverpleegkundige zorg bij veranderend beleid. NIVEL, Utrecht, 1985.

246. De vier kerndisciplines. Algemene thuiszorg gekortwiekt. Landelijk bestuurlijk overleg. Bunnik, 1986.

247. de Vries PH, de Vries Robbe PF. An overview of medical expert systems. Methods of Information in Medicine 1985; 24: 57-64.

248. Wade DT, Hewer RL. Why admit stroke patients to hospital? Lancet 1983; 1: 807-809.

249. Walker A. Meeting the needs of Canada's elderly with limited health resources: some observations based on British experience. Presented to the Colloquium on Aging with Limited Health Resources, Winnipeg, Canada, 5-6 May 1986.

250. Weiler PG. Evaluation of alternatives in long-term care. American Journal of Public Health 1983; 73: 637-639.

251. Weiss M, Worthington PH, Prioleau M, Rosato FE. Home total parenteral nutrition in cancer patients. Cancer 1982; 51: 1210-1213.

252. Wijkel D. Lower referral rates for integrated health centres in the Netherlands. Health Policy, 1986; 6: 185-198.

253. Wijkel D. Encouraging the development of integrated health centres: a critical analysis of lower referral rates. Social Science & Medicine 1986; 23: 35-41.

254. de Witte L, Van de Horst F, Joosten J, Philipsen H. Continuiteit van zorg na ontslag uit een revalidatiecentrum. Tijdschrift voor Sociale Gezondheidszorg 1986; 64: 567-572.

255. Wood P. Impairment, disability, handicap: toward the development of a functional information system. New York: World Rehabilitation Fund, 1983.

256. World Health Organization. Regional Office for Europe. Self-help and health in Europe. Copenhagen: The World Health Organization, 1983.

257. Yu VL. Conceptual obstacles in computerized medical diagnosis. Journal of Medicine and Philosophy 1983; 8: 67-75.

258. Zilz DA. Current trends in home health care. American Journal of Hospital Pharmacy 1985; 42: 2520-2525.

259. Zimmer JG, Groth-Juncker A, McCusker J. Effects of a physician-led home care team on terminal care. Journal of the American Geriatric Society 1984; 32: 288-292.

260. Zimmer JG, Groth-Juncker A, McCusker J. A randomized controlled study of a home health care team. American Journal of Public Health 1985; 75: 134-141.

261. Zimmet P. Gerstman M, Raper LR, Cohen M, Crosbie C, Kuykendall V, Michaels D, Hartmann K. Computerized assessment of self-

monitored blood glucose results using a Glucometer reflectance photometer with memory and microcomputer. Diabetes Research and Clinical Practice 1985; 1: 55-63.

262. Zomerdijk JC. Diagnostic applications of monoclonal antibodies. A report issued to the Steering Committee on Future Health Scenarios. The Hague: CIVI, 1986.

APPENDIX E ACKNOWLEDGEMENTS

Dr. Peter Groenewegen of NIVEL prepared a paper for the project on the present system of home care in the Netherlands that was the basis for Section 2 of the report. The project is very grateful to Dr. Groenewegen for this assistance. «PG»«LS1»

Working Group on The Present Home Care System in the Netherlands (June 1987)

Ing. J.J. Alexander
Innovatie Onderzoek
Programma Hulpmiddelen Gehandicapten
Maarssen

Prof. dr. ir. J.E.W. Beneken
Technische Universiteit Eindhoven
Eindhoven

Mw. mr. M.B.E.G. Brenninkmeijer
Ministerie van WVC
Rijswijk

De heer A. Dekker
NIVEL
Utrecht

Prof. dr. J.M.C. Douze
Rijksuniversiteit Utrecht
Utrecht

Prof. dr. J.C. van Es
Medisch Contact
KNMG Utrecht

Mw. Drs. M. Leemeijer
Rijksuniversiteit Groningen
Groningen

Mw. H. van der Poel
Dalfsen

Dr. D. Post
Regionaal Ziekenfonds
Zwolle

Dr. A.J.B.I Sips
Arts
Vught

Mw. M.K. Visser
Centrale Raad v. Gezinsverzorging
Driebergen

Dr. A. Vrij
Geneeskundige Hoofdinspectie
Rijswijk

Dr. L. Wierda
Ziekenfonds Amsterdam
Amsterdam

Mw. V. Wittenberg
Vrije Universiteit
Amsterdam

Prof. dr. G. Zilvold
TH Twente
Enschede

Working Group on Home Care Technology (June 1987)

Ing. J.J. Alexander
Innovatie Onderzoek
Programma Hulpmiddelen Gehandicapten
Maarssen

Prof. dr. ir. J.H. van Bemmel
Academisch Ziekenhuis V.U.
Vakgroep Medische Informatica
Amsterdam

Prof. dr. ir. J.E.W. Beneken
Technische Universiteit Eindhoven
Eindhoven

Prof. dr. H. Bouma
Technische Universiteit Eindhoven
Eindhoven

De heer A. Dekker
NIVEL
Utrecht

Prof. dr. J.M.C. Douze
Rijksuniversiteit Utrecht
Utrecht

Ing. F.G. de Graaff
Gemeenschappelijke Medische Dienst
Amsterdam

Ir. J.A.M. Graafmans
Technische Universiteit Eindhoven
Eindhoven

Ir. W.H. Leliveld
Technische Universiteit Eindhoven
Eindhoven

Mw. H. van der Poel
Dalfsen

Prof. dr. H. Schneider
Vrije Universiteit
Amsterdam

A number of other experts also commented on the draft versions of the report.

Prof. dr. H. Bakker
Vrije Universiteit
Amsterdam

S.I.M. Bless
Projekt Gezondheidszorg Almere
Almere

Mr. drs. J.P. Dopheide
Ministerie van WVC (afd. Voorzieningen Eerstelijnsgezondheidszorg)
Rijswijk

Dr. C.P. Dubbelman
Revalidatiearts
Amsterdam

Prof. dr. J.H.P. Jonxis
Haren (Gn)

Dr. C.P.M. Knipscheer
Vrije Universiteit
Amsterdam

W.P. Kramer
van Luyken Adviesbureau
Bloemendaal

A. Roeloffzen
Algemene thuiszorg in samenwerking (ATIS)
Bunnik

Dr. G. Schrijvers
Rijksuniversiteit Utrecht
Utrecht

L. Sweerts
Algemene thuiszorg in samenwerking (ATIS)
Bunnik

GPSR Compliance

The European Union's (EU) General Product Safety Regulation (GPSR) is a set of rules that requires consumer products to be safe and our obligations to ensure this.

If you have any concerns about our products, you can contact us on ProductSafety@springernature.com

In case Publisher is established outside the EU, the EU authorized representative is:

Springer Nature Customer Service Center GmbH
Europaplatz 3
69115 Heidelberg, Germany

Batch number: 10607330

Printed by Printforce, the Netherlands